The Ultimate Guide to Tourette Syndrome

Understanding and Managing the Condition

A Guide for patients, families and professionals

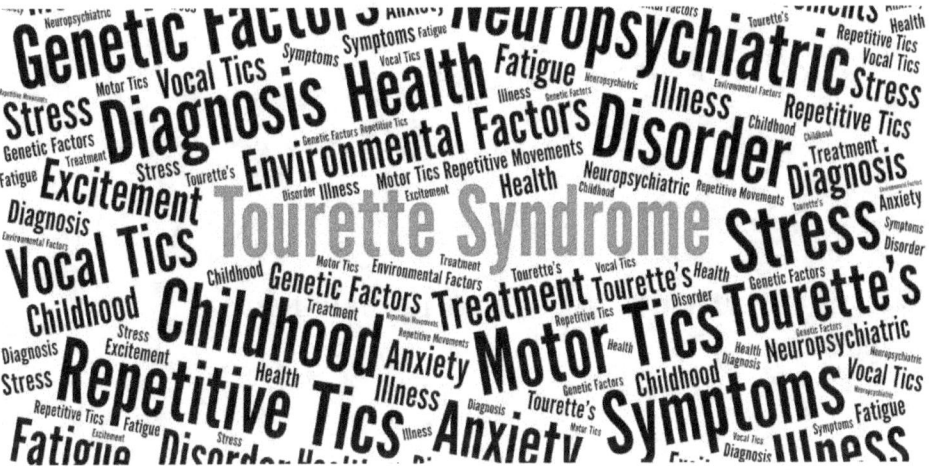

In this book, we explore the complexities of Tourette Syndrome and the impact it has on individuals and families. Through a series of questions and answers, we delve into the causes, symptoms, and treatments of TS, dispelling common misconceptions and offering hope for those affected.

We begin by examining the neurological roots of TS and how it affects the brain's functioning. We then discuss the various symptoms of TS, including motor and vocal tics, and how they can impact daily life. We also explore the different types of TS, including the lesser-known forms such as Coprolalia and Echolalia.

Next, we turn to the topic of treatment, discussing the various options available, including medication, therapy, and lifestyle changes. We examine the pros and cons of each approach and offer guidance on how to work with healthcare professionals to find the best course of treatment.

In addition to medical interventions, we also explore the role of mindfulness and self-care in managing TS. We discuss the benefits of practices such as meditation, yoga, and deep breathing, and offer tips for incorporating these activities into daily life. We highlight the importance of awareness and understanding, and offer practical advice for families, educators, and healthcare professionals on how to support individuals with TS.

Ultimately, this book aims to provide a comprehensive guide to Tourette Syndrome, empowering readers with knowledge, hope, and a deeper understanding of this complex and often misunderstood condition.

Table of Contents

Introduction

What is Tourette Syndrome (TS)?

Tourette syndrome, often abbreviated as TS, represents a complex neurological disorder with a constellation of features that encompass simple and complex motor tics, vocal tics, and sometimes, obsessive-compulsive symptoms. This condition typically makes its debut in individuals before they reach the age of 2 A hallmark of TS is its waxing and waning course, although it is not uncommon for tics to persist into adulthood, underscoring the chronic nature of the disorder. It is intriguing to note that TS primarily manifests in males, lending credence to a genetic component with varying degrees of expression or penetrance.

The underlying pathological mechanism governing Tourette syndrome remains somewhat elusive, yet a plethora of research has provided valuable insights into its etiology. Neuroanatomical studies, coupled with neuroimaging techniques, have offered a glimpse into the intricate workings of the brain in individuals with TS. Additionally, the therapeutic landscape has been shaped by the effectiveness of antipsychotic medications, hinting at the involvement of the dopaminergic system in the basal ganglia as a pivotal player in the pathogenesis of TS.

Central to the understanding of TS is the discussion of causative mechanisms that disrupt dopaminergic neurotransmission. Among these mechanisms, a noteworthy contender is the notion of an infection-triggered inflammatory immune process. It is not without precedent in the realm of neurology that extrapyramidal movement disorders can manifest as a consequence of post-streptococcal infections, exemplified by conditions like Sydenham's chorea. In light of these observations, it has been proposed that some cases of childhood-onset TS may be rooted in a post-streptococcal mechanism, contributing to a broader spectrum of childhood neurobehavioral disorders collectively labeled as Pediatric Autoimmune Neuropsychiatric Disorder Associated with Streptococcal Infection (PANDAS).

The convergence of TS and PANDAS has been a subject of intense scrutiny within the medical community, prompting a critical examination of the PANDAS concept itself. This complex interplay between TS and PANDAS underscores the multifaceted nature of these disorders, which demands a nuanced approach to diagnosis and treatment. Indeed, understanding the various pathological mechanisms at play is essential, as it not only hinges on the distinction between acute and chronic infections but also considers the autoimmune processes that may underlie the conditions.

In light of these considerations, the therapeutic armamentarium for TS encompasses a wide array of strategies. Typical and atypical antipsychotic medications have been cornerstones of treatment, offering relief from the often distressing symptoms. Moreover, experimental therapies such as repetitive transcranial magnetic stimulation and deep brain stimulation have garnered attention for their potential to ameliorate the symptoms of TS. The choice of therapeutic approach should be meticulously considered in light of the individual's unique clinical presentation and the underlying pathological processes at play.

Tourette syndrome is a multifaceted neurological disorder characterized by a combination of motor and vocal tics, often accompanied by obsessive-compulsive symptoms. While the precise pathological mechanisms remain a subject of ongoing research, the disturbance of the dopaminergic system in the basal ganglia has emerged as a key player. The intersection of TS with PANDAS adds complexity to the diagnostic and therapeutic landscape, necessitating a thorough understanding of the interplay between infection-triggered immune processes and autoimmunity. As we delve deeper into the complexities of TS, a more refined approach to diagnosis and treatment will continue to evolve, offering hope to those affected by this condition.

History of TS

The history of Tourette syndrome (TS) is a compelling journey through time, marked by a quest to comprehend the enigmatic nature of this neurological disorder. TS, characterized by motor and vocal tics, often accompanied by obsessive-compulsive symptoms, has been recognized and studied for centuries, though its understanding has evolved significantly.

Early Observations

The earliest documented cases of individuals exhibiting symptoms resembling TS date back to the 15th century. In 1489, a French physician named Gilles de la Tourette provided one of the earliest descriptions of the syndrome. However, it wasn't until the late 19th century that more systematic and detailed observations were made.

Jean-Martin Charcot and Georges Gilles de la Tourette

It was in the late 19th century that the disorder gained substantial recognition, largely due to the work of the renowned French neurologist Jean-Martin Charcot. Charcot's student and colleague, Georges Gilles de la Tourette, made significant contributions by providing comprehensive clinical descriptions of patients exhibiting the characteristic tics and verbal outbursts.

Early Nomenclature

Initially, the disorder was referred to as "maladie des tics" or "tic maladie." However, in 1885, Gilles de la Tourette published a comprehensive study on the subject, and the eponymous term "Gilles de la Tourette syndrome" came into existence. This name has persisted in the medical literature.

Recognition in the 20th Century

The 20th century saw a growing interest in TS, with researchers delving into the neurological underpinnings of the disorder. Neuroimaging studies and advancements in psychology shed light on the complex interplay between the brain and TS symptoms. It became increasingly clear that TS was not simply a behavioral issue but had neurological roots.

Advances in Treatment

In the latter half of the 20th century, treatment options for TS started to expand. Antipsychotic medications, such as haloperidol and pimozide, were found to be effective in managing tics. Additionally, behavioral therapies and support groups became important components of treatment for individuals with TS.

Recognition as a Spectrum

The understanding of TS evolved to encompass a broader spectrum of tic-related disorders, acknowledging that not all cases were as severe or disabling as the classic presentation. This recognition led to a more comprehensive understanding of the syndrome and improved diagnostic criteria.

Genetic and Neurological Insights

Advances in genetics and neuroscience in the late 20th and early 21st centuries shed further light on TS. Research indicated that there was a hereditary component, and specific genetic markers were identified. Neuroimaging studies demonstrated the involvement of the basal ganglia and dopaminergic pathways.

Contemporary Research and Future Directions

Research into TS continues to this day, with a focus on uncovering the precise neurological mechanisms and potential new treatments. Genetic studies, neuroimaging techniques, and a better understanding of the immune system's role in TS have contributed to our evolving comprehension of the disorder.

The history of Tourette syndrome is a story of progression from early, vague observations to a more refined and comprehensive understanding of the disorder. While its origins date back centuries, it was the work of 19th-century pioneers and subsequent research that elevated TS to a recognized neurological condition. Today, ongoing research endeavors offer hope for continued progress in the diagnosis and treatment of TS, ultimately improving the lives of those affected by this complex disorder.

Prevalence and epidemiology of TS

Tourette syndrome (TS) is a neurodevelopmental disorder characterized by multiple motor tics and at least one vocal tic, often involving repetitive movements or sounds. The prevalence and epidemiology of TS have been studied extensively in recent years, and here are some key findings

Prevalence TS is estimated to affect approximately 1% of children and adolescents worldwide, with a male-to-female ratio of about 2 In adults, the prevalence of TS is thought to be around 0.6%.

Incidence The incidence of TS is highest during childhood, with most cases appearing between the ages of 5 and 1 The peak age of onset is typically around 7-10 years old.

Familial risk TS tends to run in families, with studies suggesting that individuals with a family history of TS are more likely to develop the disorder themselves. The risk is higher if the family member has a severe form of TS.

Genetic mutations Several genetic mutations have been identified as risk factors for TS, including those affecting the dopamine receptor D2 (DRD2), the dopamine transporter (DAT), and the serotonin transporter (SERT). However, it's important to note that genetics alone do not guarantee the development of TS, and environmental factors may also play a role.

Comorbidities Individuals with TS often have co-occurring conditions, such as attention deficit hyperactivity disorder (ADHD), obsessive-compulsive disorder (OCD), anxiety disorders, and depression.

Ethnicity TS appears to affect all ethnic groups equally, although there may be variations in how TS presents itself across different cultures.

Socioeconomic status There is no clear association between socioeconomic status and the development of TS.

Geographic location There is no evidence to suggest that TS is more common in certain geographic locations.

Urban vs. rural Some studies suggest that TS may be more common in urban areas, possibly due to increased exposure to environmental stressors or improved access to healthcare services. Access to care Despite advances in our understanding of TS, many individuals with the disorder still face challenges in accessing appropriate medical care, particularly in underserved communities.

These findings provide a snapshot of the prevalence and epidemiology of Tourette syndrome. It's essential to remember that each individual with TS is unique, and their specific needs and experiences may vary from those of others with the disorder.

Myth vs. reality about TS

To start, it's important to distinguish between myths and realities about TS. Here are some common misconceptions and facts about TS

Myth TS is a mental illness.

Reality TS is a neurodevelopmental disorder, not a mental illness. It is characterized by multiple motor tics and at least one vocal tic, which can be involuntary sounds or words.

Myth People with TS are unable to control their tics.

Reality While people with TS may not be able to completely control their tics, they often have some degree of control over them. Many people with TS can suppress their tics to some extent, especially in situations where they feel anxious or self-conscious.

Myth TS is caused by poor parenting or a stressful environment.

Reality There is no scientific evidence to support this claim. TS is thought to be caused by a combination of genetic and environmental factors, but the exact cause is still unknown.

Myth People with TS are less intelligent or capable than others.

Reality TS does not affect intelligence or cognitive ability. In fact, many people with TS are highly intelligent and successful in their fields.

Myth TS is rare.

Reality TS is more common than previously thought. According to the National Institute of Neurological Disorders and Stroke, TS affects an estimated 200,000 people in the United States, and it is estimated that 1 in 160 children between the ages of 5 and 17 have TS.

Myth TS can be cured with medication or therapy.

Reality While there is no cure for TS, various treatments can help manage symptoms. Medications such as dopamine blockers and antipsychotics can help reduce tic severity, and therapies like habit reversal training and exposure and response prevention can also be effective.

Myth People with TS are all the same.

Reality Every person with TS is unique, and their experiences and symptoms can vary greatly. It's important to avoid making assumptions about people with TS and to treat each person as an individual.

It's important to be respectful and understanding when discussing TS, and to rely on credible sources of information. If you have any further questions or concerns, feel free to ask!

Chapter 1

Causes and Genetics of Tourette Syndrome

What are the known causes of TS?

The exact causes of Tourette Syndrome (TS) are not yet fully understood, but research suggests that it is a complex interplay of genetic, environmental, and neurochemical factors. Here are some of the known causes and contributing factors

Genetics TS tends to run in families, and several genes have been identified as potential risk factors. However, no single gene is responsible for causing TS, and the inheritance pattern is thought to be multifactorial.

Brain structure and function People with TS tend to have differences in brain structure and function, particularly in areas responsible for movement, motor control, and cognition. These differences may contribute to the development of tics.

Neurotransmitters Imbalances in neurotransmitters such as dopamine, serotonin, and gamma-aminobutyric acid (GABA) have been linked to TS. These chemicals play a role in regulating movement, mood, and other functions that are affected in TS.

Environmental factors Stress, anxiety, and other environmental factors can trigger or exacerbate tics in people with TS. Infections, allergies, and other medical conditions can also contribute to the development of tics.

Autoimmune disorders Some research suggests that TS may be linked to autoimmune disorders, in which the immune system mistakenly attacks healthy cells and tissues in the body.

Other factors Sleep disorders, anxiety disorders, and attention deficit hyperactivity disorder (ADHD) are common in people with TS. These conditions may contribute to the development of tics or make them worse.

It's important to note that TS is a complex condition, and no single factor can fully explain its causes. Each person with TS may have a unique combination of risk factors and contributing conditions that contribute to their tics and other symptoms.

Here are some additional facts that you may find interesting

Tourette Syndrome is not just about tics While tics are the most visible symptom of TS, they are not the only symptom. Many people with TS also experience other neurological symptoms, such as attention deficit hyperactivity disorder (ADHD), obsessive-compulsive disorder (OCD), and anxiety disorders.

TS is a spectrum disorder TS is not a single disorder, but rather a spectrum of disorders. There are different types of tics, and people with TS can experience a range of symptoms, from mild to severe.

TS is not caused by poor self-control Contrary to popular belief, TS is not caused by a lack of self-control or willpower. Tics are involuntary movements that are beyond the control of the individual.

TS can be treated with deep brain stimulation In some cases, TS can be treated with deep brain stimulation, a surgical procedure that involves implanting an electrode in the brain to deliver electrical impulses to specific areas.

TS is not a result of poor parenting TS is not caused by poor parenting or a dysfunctional family environment. It is a neurological disorder that can affect anyone, regardless of their upbringing or family background.

TS can be managed with medication There are several medications that can be used to manage the symptoms of TS, including dopamine blockers, antipsychotics, and antidepressants.

TS can be mistaken for other disorders TS can be mistaken for other disorders, such as ADHD, OCD, or anxiety disorders. It is important to receive a proper diagnosis from a qualified healthcare professional.

TS can affect anyone TS can affect anyone, regardless of age, gender, or ethnicity. It is estimated that approximately 1 in 160 children between the ages of 5 and 17 have TS.

TS has a significant impact on quality of life TS can have a significant impact on a person's quality of life, affecting their social, emotional, and academic functioning.

TS is not something to be ashamed of TS is a neurological disorder, and it is not something to be ashamed of. People with TS are not weak or flawed, and they deserve the same respect and dignity as anyone else.

What is the role of genetics in TS?

The role of genetics in Tourette Syndrome (TS) is not fully understood, but research suggests that genetic factors play a significant role in the development of the disorder.

TS is known to run in families, and studies have found that individuals with a family history of TS are more likely to develop the disorder themselves. However, the inheritance pattern of TS is complex, and it is not clear how genetic factors contribute to the development of the disorder.

Several genes have been identified as potential risk factors for TS, including genes involved in the regulation of dopamine and serotonin, two neurotransmitters that play a role in movement and motor control. Some of these genes include

Dopamine receptor D2 (DRD2) gene The DRD2 gene has been associated with TS, and certain variations in this gene have been found to increase the risk of developing the disorder.

Dopamine transporter (DAT) gene The DAT gene has also been linked to TS, and variations in this gene have been found to affect the function of dopamine in the brain.

Serotonin transporter (SERT) gene The SERT gene has been associated with TS, and variations in this gene have been found to affect the function of serotonin in the brain.

MTHFR gene The MTHFR gene is involved in the metabolism of homocysteine, an amino acid that is important for the function of dopamine and serotonin. Certain variations in the MTHFR gene have been found to increase the risk of developing TS.

While genetic factors are thought to play a role in the development of TS, it is important to note that genetics alone do not determine whether someone will develop the disorder. Environmental factors, such as stress and other psychological factors, can also contribute to the development of TS.

There is currently no genetic test available to diagnose TS, and diagnosis is typically made based on a combination of clinical evaluation and behavioral observations. However, genetic research may lead to the development of new treatments and therapies for TS in the future.

What are the latest advances in TS research?

The neurobiological underpinnings of Tourette syndrome (TS) are complex and multifaceted, and research has explored various neurotransmitters, environmental factors, and psychological elements in relation to this condition.

Neurotransmitters in TS

While dopamine dysfunction within the basal ganglia is widely recognized as a key factor in TS, other neurotransmitters have also been investigated. Some of these include

Serotonin (5-HT) Imbalances in serotonin transmission have been linked to TS. This is particularly relevant as medications targeting serotonin, such as selective serotonin reuptake inhibitors (SSRIs), have been used to manage co-occurring symptoms, like obsessive-compulsive disorder (OCD), which often accompanies TS.

Gamma-Aminobutyric Acid (GABA) GABA, the primary inhibitory neurotransmitter in the brain, has also been implicated in TS. Some research suggests that GABAergic dysfunction may contribute to the motor and vocal tics observed in TS.

Glutamate Glutamate is the primary excitatory neurotransmitter in the brain. Imbalances in glutamatergic signaling may play a role in TS, as suggested by some studies. This opens avenues for exploring treatments targeting glutamate receptors.

Environmental Factors Contributing to TS

TS is considered a complex interplay of genetic and environmental factors. Several environmental elements have been proposed as potential contributors to the development or exacerbation of TS

Infections There is evidence to suggest that certain infections, especially streptococcal infections, may trigger or worsen tics in some individuals. This aligns with the concept of Pediatric Autoimmune Neuropsychiatric Disorder Associated with Streptococcal Infection (PANDAS), which links streptococcal infections to the onset or exacerbation of tics and related symptoms.

Prenatal and Perinatal Factors Adverse prenatal or perinatal events, such as maternal smoking during pregnancy, premature birth, or low birth weight, have been investigated for potential links to the development of TS.

Psychosocial Stress While the exact relationship between stress and TS remains complex, stress and psychosocial factors are believed to exacerbate tic symptoms. The experience of tics can be stressful, and the social consequences of the condition can also contribute to elevated stress levels.

Psychological Factors and TS

The relationship between psychological factors and TS is intricate

Psychological Stress Stress can exacerbate tics in individuals with TS. The experience of living with tics, especially in social situations, can be stressful, creating a feedback loop where stress worsens tics, and tics, in turn, create more stress.

Psychiatric Comorbidities Individuals with TS often experience psychiatric comorbidities, such as OCD, attention-deficit/hyperactivity disorder (ADHD), and anxiety. These conditions can contribute to psychological stress and complicate the clinical picture.

Coping Mechanisms Psychological factors can also influence the use of coping mechanisms. Some individuals with TS develop strategies to manage their tics or mask them in social situations, which can have psychological consequences.

The etiology of Tourette syndrome is multifaceted. While dopamine dysfunction is a key player, other neurotransmitters, such as serotonin, GABA, and glutamate, also contribute to the neurological underpinnings of TS. Environmental factors, including infections and prenatal/perinatal events, have been explored in relation to the development of TS. Additionally, psychological stress and psychiatric comorbidities can both exacerbate and be exacerbated by TS symptoms, making it imperative for a holistic approach in understanding and managing this complex disorder.

Chapter 2

Symptoms and Diagnosis of Tourette Syndrome

What are the different types of tics?

Tics are sudden, recurring movements or sounds that are commonly associated with Tourette Syndrome (TS). There are several different types of tics, including

Motor tics These are sudden, involuntary movements or contractions of a muscle or a group of muscles. Motor tics can be simple or complex. Simple motor tics include movements such as blinking, facial grimacing, head jerking, or arm or leg movements. Complex motor tics include coordinated movements such as touching, rubbing, or tapping certain body parts, or performing a sequence of movements.

Vocal tics These are sudden, involuntary sounds or words that are uttered without intent. Vocal tics can be simple or complex. Simple vocal tics include sounds such as grunting, sniffing, or clearing the throat. Complex vocal tics include words or phrases that are repeated, such as coprolalia (the repeated use of obscene words) or echolalia (the repeated use of words or phrases heard previously).

Tic-like behaviors These are movements or sounds that resemble tics but are not necessarily involuntary. Tic-like behaviors can include habits such as nail biting, hair twirling, or foot tapping.

Stereotypies These are repetitive, purposeless movements that are often seen in individuals with autism spectrum disorder or other developmental disorders. Stereotypies can include hand flapping, arm waving, or body rocking.

Mannerisms These are habitual, involuntary movements or postures that are often seen in individuals with TS. Mannerisms can include twirling hair, tapping feet, or adjusting clothing.

Coping mechanisms These are behaviors that individuals with TS may use to manage their tics or other symptoms. Coping mechanisms can include activities such as pacing, fidgeting, or engaging in repetitive behaviors.

It's important to note that tics can vary in severity, frequency, and type over time, and may change in response to stress, anxiety, or other environmental factors.

Common Coping Mechanisms for Individuals with TS

Individuals with Tourette syndrome (TS) often develop coping strategies to manage their tics and the social challenges they may face. These coping mechanisms can vary widely from person to person and may include

1. **Tic Suppression** Some individuals with TS learn to suppress their tics temporarily. This involves consciously holding back or delaying the expression of a tic when in public or during situations where it might be socially disruptive. However, tic suppression can be mentally and physically exhausting.

2. **Substitution** In some cases, individuals with TS develop "acceptable" or less noticeable movements or sounds to substitute for their tics. These substitutions can be less disruptive and socially acceptable.

3. **Environmental Avoidance** People with TS may avoid environments or situations that trigger their tics. For example, if a loud, crowded place exacerbates their tics, they might choose to avoid such settings.

4. **Awareness and Relaxation Techniques** Mindfulness and relaxation techniques can help individuals become more aware of their tics and reduce their intensity. Techniques like deep breathing, progressive muscle relaxation, and biofeedback can be helpful.

5. **Support Groups and Counseling** Support groups provide individuals with TS a platform to share their experiences, learn from others, and gain emotional support. Counseling or therapy, such as cognitive-behavioral therapy, can help individuals manage the emotional and psychological aspects of TS.

6. **Medication** In cases where tics are particularly severe or interfering with daily life, medication may be prescribed. Antipsychotic medications, such as haloperidol or aripiprazole, can help reduce tic severity. However, the decision to use medication is typically made after careful consideration of potential side effects and individual circumstances.

Environmental Triggers for Tics

Tics in TS can be influenced by environmental factors, though the relationship between specific triggers and tics is complex and varies from person to person. Some common environmental factors that may trigger tics include

1. **Stress and Anxiety** Emotional stress and anxiety can exacerbate tics in many individuals with TS. High-stress situations, such as public speaking or exams, often lead to an increase in tics.

2. **Excitement or Anticipation** Positive emotions like excitement or anticipation can also trigger tics in some cases. For example, someone may experience an increase in tics before a fun event.

3. **Social Pressure** Social situations, especially those where an individual feels observed or judged, can lead to heightened tic activity. The effort to suppress tics in these situations may intensify them.

4. **Temperature and Humidity** Some individuals with TS find that changes in temperature and humidity can affect their tics. Extreme heat or cold may trigger increased tic activity.

5. **Fatigue and Illness** Being fatigued or having an illness may make tics more pronounced, as the body's resources for suppressing tics become depleted.

Treatments and Therapies for Managing Tics

Several treatments and therapies are available to help manage tics in individuals with TS

1. **Behavioral Therapies** Behavioral therapies like Habit Reversal Training (HRT) and Comprehensive Behavioral Intervention for Tics (CBIT) are designed to help individuals become more aware of their tics and develop strategies to manage and reduce them.

2. **Medications** Antipsychotic medications, including haloperidol, risperidone, and aripiprazole, can be prescribed to reduce the severity of tics. These medications are often considered when tics significantly impair daily functioning.

3. **Repetitive Transcranial Magnetic Stimulation (rTMS)** rTMS is a non-invasive technique that uses magnetic fields to stimulate specific brain areas. Some studies have explored its potential for reducing tic severity in TS.

4. **Deep Brain Stimulation (DBS)** DBS is an invasive procedure that involves implanting electrodes in the brain to modulate abnormal neural activity. It may be considered in severe cases of TS when other treatments are ineffective.

5. **Supportive Therapies** Support groups, counseling, and psychotherapy can help individuals and their families cope with the emotional and psychological aspects of TS.

The choice of treatment or therapy depends on the severity of tics, the individual's specific needs, and their response to interventions. A comprehensive and individualized approach is essential for managing tics and improving the quality of life for those with TS.

How is TS diagnosed?

Tourette Syndrome (TS) can be diagnosed by a qualified healthcare professional, such as a neurologist, psychiatrist, or a pediatrician, based on a combination of clinical evaluation, medical history, and behavioral observations. Here are the steps involved in diagnosing TS

Medical history The healthcare professional will ask questions about the individual's medical history, including any previous diagnoses, medications, and surgeries. They will also ask about the individual's family medical history, including any history of TS or other neurodevelopmental disorders.

Physical examination The healthcare professional will perform a physical examination to rule out any other medical conditions that may be causing or contributing to the tics. They may check for muscle weakness, balance problems, or other signs of neurological dysfunction.

Neurological examination The healthcare professional may perform a neurological examination to check for signs of neurological dysfunction, such as abnormal reflexes, muscle weakness, or sensory problems.

Behavioral observations The healthcare professional will observe the individual's behavior and tics to determine their severity, frequency, and duration. They may use standardized tools, such as the Yale Global Tic Severity Scale or the Tic Severity Scale, to assess the severity of the tics.

Psychiatric evaluation The healthcare professional may perform a psychiatric evaluation to rule out other psychiatric conditions, such as anxiety or depression, that may be contributing to the tics. They may use standardized tools, such as the Mental Health Clinician's Interview or the Structured Clinical Interview for DSM-IV, to assess the individual's mental health.

Genetic testing Genetic testing may be recommended to rule out other genetic disorders that may be causing or contributing to the tics.

Imaging studies Imaging studies, such as magnetic resonance imaging (MRI) or computerized tomography (CT) scans, may be ordered to rule out other neurological conditions, such as a stroke or a tumor, that may be causing the tics.

Diagnostic criteria The healthcare professional will use the diagnostic criteria for TS, which are outlined in the Diagnostic and Statistical Manual of Mental Disorders, 5th Edition (DSM-5), to determine if the individual's symptoms meet the criteria for TS.

It's important to note that TS can be difficult to diagnose, as it can resemble other conditions, such as attention deficit hyperactivity disorder (ADHD) or anxiety disorders. A comprehensive evaluation by a qualified healthcare professional is necessary to accurately diagnose TS.

Tourette Syndrome (TS) is a neurodevelopmental disorder characterized by multiple motor tics and at least one vocal tic. Motor tics are sudden, involuntary movements or contractions of a muscle or a group of muscles, while vocal tics are sounds or words that are repeated over and over again.

The exact cause of TS is not known, but it is believed to be related to abnormalities in certain areas of the brain, including the basal ganglia and the cortex. The disorder tends to run in families, and there is evidence that genetics play a role in its development.

The symptoms of TS can vary widely from person to person, and they may change over time. Motor tics can be simple or complex, and they can affect any part of the body. Simple motor tics include things like blinking, facial grimacing, head jerking, or arm or leg movements. Complex motor tics can involve coordinated movements, such as touching or rubbing certain body parts, or performing a sequence of movements.

Vocal tics are also a common symptom of TS. They can be simple, such as grunting, sniffing, or clearing the throat, or they can be complex, such as repeating words or phrases. In some cases, vocal tics can be obscene or inappropriate, which can be distressing for the individual and their family.

TS can also be associated with other conditions, such as attention deficit hyperactivity disorder (ADHD), obsessive-compulsive disorder (OCD), and anxiety disorders. These conditions can make it difficult for individuals with TS to function in daily life, and they may require additional treatment.

There is no cure for TS, but there are several treatments available that can help manage the symptoms. Behavioral therapies, such as habit reversal training and exposure and response prevention, can help individuals with TS reduce their tics. Medications, such as dopamine blockers and antipsychotics, can also be effective in reducing tics, but they can have side effects. In some cases, deep brain stimulation may be recommended, which involves implanting a device that delivers electrical impulses to the brain to help regulate tics.

It's important to note that TS is not a result of poor self-control or a person's upbringing or environment. It is a neurological disorder that requires understanding and support from family, friends, and healthcare professionals. With appropriate treatment and support, individuals with TS can lead fulfilling lives and achieve their goals.

Common Symptoms of Tourette Syndrome (TS)

Tourette Syndrome is characterized by the presence of motor tics (involuntary movements) and vocal tics (involuntary sounds or vocalizations). Some common symptoms of TS include

1. **Motor Tics** These are repetitive, sudden, and often rapid movements that can involve various parts of the body. Common motor tics include blinking, head jerking, facial grimacing, shoulder shrugging, and repetitive tapping.

2. **Vocal Tics** Vocal tics are involuntary sounds or words produced by the individual. They can range from throat clearing, grunting, and sniffing to more complex vocalizations, such as repeating words or phrases. Coprolalia, which involves involuntary swearing or inappropriate comments, is a rare but well-known vocal tic associated with TS.

3. **Complex Tics** Complex tics involve a combination of motor and vocal elements. For example, a person with TS might have a motor tic like touching their nose followed by a vocal tic like making a specific noise.

4. **Premonitory Urge** Many individuals with TS experience a premonitory urge before the expression of tics. These are uncomfortable sensations or feelings that precede the tics and are temporarily relieved by performing the tic. For some, suppressing these urges can be distressing.

5. **Waxing and Waning Course** TS often exhibits a waxing and waning course, where the severity and frequency of tics can fluctuate over time. Tics may temporarily improve or worsen.

6. **Onset in Childhood** TS typically emerges in childhood, with the most common age of onset occurring between 5 and 10 years old. The initial tics are usually simple motor or vocal tics.

7. **Comorbid Conditions** TS often co-occurs with other conditions, such as Attention-Deficit/Hyperactivity Disorder (ADHD), Obsessive-Compulsive Disorder (OCD), anxiety disorders, and depression.

Treatments for Tourette Syndrome

The management of Tourette Syndrome is individualized, and treatment options are tailored to the specific needs of the person with TS. Some common treatments include

1. **Behavioral Therapies** Behavioral therapies, such as Habit Reversal Training (HRT) and Comprehensive Behavioral Intervention for Tics (CBIT), are designed to help individuals become more aware of their tics and develop strategies to manage and reduce them.

2. **Medications** Medications are often used to manage tics in TS, especially when they significantly impair daily functioning. Common medications include antipsychotics like haloperidol, risperidone, aripiprazole, and others. These medications can reduce the severity of tics.

3. **Repetitive Transcranial Magnetic Stimulation (rTMS)** rTMS is a non-invasive technique that uses magnetic fields to stimulate specific brain areas. Some studies have explored its potential for reducing tic severity in TS.

4. **Deep Brain Stimulation (DBS)** DBS is an invasive procedure that involves implanting electrodes in the brain to modulate abnormal neural activity. It may be considered in severe cases of TS when other treatments are ineffective.

5. **Supportive Therapies** Support groups, counseling, and psychotherapy can help individuals and their families cope with the emotional and psychological aspects of TS.

Medication for Managing TS

Medication can be an effective treatment option for managing TS, especially when tics are severe or significantly impact a person's daily life. Antipsychotic medications, such as haloperidol, risperidone, and aripiprazole, are commonly prescribed to reduce the severity of tics.

It's important to note that medication should be carefully considered, and the decision to use it should be made in consultation with a healthcare provider. Medications may have potential side effects, and the benefits of tic reduction should be weighed against these potential drawbacks.

Tourette Syndrome is characterized by motor and vocal tics that often emerge in childhood. Treatment options for TS include behavioral therapies, medications, and in some cases, more advanced interventions like rTMS and

DBS. Medication can be effective in managing tics but should be used judiciously, considering individual needs and potential side effects. An individualized approach to treatment is key to improving the quality of life for those with TS.

Common Treatments for Associated Conditions like ADHD and OCD

Individuals with Tourette Syndrome (TS) often experience co-occurring conditions like Attention-Deficit/Hyperactivity Disorder (ADHD) and Obsessive-Compulsive Disorder (OCD). Here are some common treatments for these associated conditions

For ADHD

1. **Stimulant Medications** Medications like methylphenidate and amphetamine-based drugs are often prescribed to manage the symptoms of ADHD. These medications can improve attention, focus, and impulse control.

2. **Non-Stimulant Medications** Non-stimulant medications, such as atomoxetine and guanfacine, may be considered for individuals who do not respond well to stimulants or have concerns about their use.

3. **Behavioral Therapy** Behavioral interventions, such as cognitive-behavioral therapy (CBT) and behavior modification strategies, can help individuals with ADHD develop coping skills and improve executive function.

4. **Educational Support** Educational accommodations, including Individualized Education Programs (IEPs) or 504 plans, can provide academic support for students with ADHD.

For OCD

1. **Cognitive-Behavioral Therapy (CBT)** CBT is a leading treatment for OCD. Exposure and Response Prevention (ERP) is a specific form of CBT that involves exposing individuals to their obsessions (the distressing thoughts) and preventing them from engaging in compulsive behaviors. Over time, this can help reduce the impact of OCD.

2. **Medications** Selective Serotonin Reuptake Inhibitors (SSRIs), such as fluoxetine, sertraline, and fluvoxamine, are commonly prescribed for OCD. They help regulate serotonin levels in the brain and can reduce obsessive thoughts and compulsive behaviors.

3. **Combination Therapy** In some cases, a combination of CBT and medication may be the most effective approach for managing OCD.

Support Groups and Organizations for Tourette Syndrome

Several support groups and organizations provide valuable resources and assistance for individuals and families dealing with Tourette Syndrome. Some of these include

1. **Tourette Association of America (TAA)** TAA is a leading organization dedicated to supporting individuals and families affected by TS. They offer resources, educational materials, and host events to raise awareness and provide a sense of community.

2. **Local Support Groups** Many local chapters of TAA or independent TS support groups exist across the United States. These groups offer opportunities for individuals and families to connect with others facing similar challenges.

3. **Online Communities** Online platforms and social media groups provide forums for individuals with TS and their families to share experiences, seek advice, and find emotional support.

Habit Reversal Training (HRT) and Exposure and Response Prevention (ERP)

Habit Reversal Training (HRT) Habit Reversal Training is a behavioral therapy approach often used to manage tics in individuals with Tourette Syndrome. It consists of several components

1. **Awareness Training** Individuals learn to identify when their tics are about to occur or when they experience premonitory urges, which are uncomfortable sensations preceding tics.

2. **Competing Response** In HRT, individuals are taught to develop a specific, voluntary response that is physically incompatible with their tics. For instance, if someone has a motor tic involving their shoulder, they might learn to contract the opposite shoulder muscle as a competing response.

3. **Social Support** A supportive environment and understanding from family and friends are crucial for the success of HRT.

Exposure and Response Prevention (ERP) Exposure and Response Prevention is a specialized form of Cognitive-Behavioral Therapy (CBT) used in the treatment of Obsessive-Compulsive Disorder (OCD). It involves

1. **Exposure** Individuals are gradually exposed to situations or stimuli that trigger their obsessive thoughts. This exposure is done in a controlled and systematic manner.

45

2. **Response Prevention** During exposure, individuals are prevented from engaging in their typical compulsive behaviors. This aims to break the cycle of obsessions and compulsions.

3. **Homework and Practice** Individuals often practice exposure exercises outside of therapy sessions to generalize the skills they've learned.

Both HRT and ERP are highly individualized and require the guidance of trained therapists. They can be effective in reducing tic severity in TS and alleviating the symptoms of OCD, respectively.

What are the differential diagnoses of TS?

Tourette Syndrome (TS) can be difficult to diagnose, as it can resemble other conditions. The following are some of the differential diagnoses of TS

Attention Deficit Hyperactivity Disorder (ADHD) TS can be mistaken for ADHD, as both conditions can involve impulsivity, hyperactivity, and inattention. However, ADHD does not typically involve the repetitive, involuntary movements or vocalizations that are characteristic of TS.

Obsessive-Compulsive Disorder (OCD) TS can be confused with OCD, as both conditions can involve repetitive behaviors or thoughts. However, in TS, the repetitive behaviors are typically involuntary, whereas in OCD, they are voluntary and driven by obsessive thoughts.

Anxiety Disorders TS can be mistaken for an anxiety disorder, as individuals with TS may experience anxiety or stress that can exacerbate their tics. However, TS is a distinct condition that involves involuntary movements or vocalizations, whereas anxiety disorders typically involve excessive worry or fear.

Motor Tic Disorders TS can be confused with other motor tic disorders, such as dystonia or chorea. However, TS typically involves multiple motor tics, while other motor tic disorders may involve a single tic or a few tics that are not as frequent or severe as those seen in TS.

Neurodegenerative Disorders TS can be mistaken for neurodegenerative disorders, such as Parkinson's disease or Huntington's disease, as all three conditions can involve involuntary movements. However, TS typically involves sudden, brief movements, whereas neurodegenerative disorders typically involve slower, more gradual movements.

Brain Injury or Infection TS can be confused with conditions that result from brain injury or infection, such as encephalitis or meningitis. However, TS is typically a chronic condition that develops over time, whereas conditions resulting from brain injury or infection can have a more sudden onset.

Psychogenic Disorders TS can be mistaken for psychogenic disorders, such as factitious disorder or conversion disorder, as individuals with TS may experience psychological distress or conversion symptoms. However, TS is a neurological condition that involves involuntary movements or vocalizations, whereas psychogenic disorders are driven by psychological factors.

Somatic Symptom Disorder TS can be confused with somatic symptom disorder, as individuals with TS may experience physical symptoms such as pain or fatigue. However, TS is a neurological condition that involves involuntary movements or vocalizations, whereas somatic symptom disorder is a psychological condition that involves excessive thoughts or concerns about physical symptoms.

It's important to note that TS can co-occur with other conditions, and a thorough diagnostic evaluation is necessary to rule out other potential causes of the symptoms.

Common Symptoms of Tourette Syndrome (TS)

1. **Motor Tics** These are repetitive, sudden, and often rapid movements that can involve various parts of the body. Common motor tics include blinking, head jerking, facial grimacing, shoulder shrugging, and repetitive tapping.

2. **Vocal Tics** Vocal tics are involuntary sounds or words produced by the individual. They can range from throat clearing, grunting, and sniffing to more complex vocalizations, such as repeating words or phrases. Coprolalia, which involves involuntary swearing or inappropriate comments, is a rare but well-known vocal tic associated with TS.

3. **Complex Tics** Complex tics involve a combination of motor and vocal elements. For example, a person with TS might have a motor tic like touching their nose followed by a vocal tic like making a specific noise.

4. **Premonitory Urge** Many individuals with TS experience a premonitory urge before the expression of tics. These are uncomfortable sensations or feelings that precede the tics and are temporarily relieved by performing the tic. For some, suppressing these urges can be distressing.

5. **Waxing and Waning Course** TS often exhibits a waxing and waning course, where the severity and frequency of tics can fluctuate over time. Tics may temporarily improve or worsen.

6. **Onset in Childhood** TS typically emerges in childhood, with the most common age of onset occurring between 5 and 10 years old. The initial tics are usually simple motor or vocal tics.

7. **Comorbid Conditions** TS often co-occurs with other conditions, such as Attention-Deficit/Hyperactivity Disorder (ADHD), Obsessive-Compulsive Disorder (OCD), anxiety disorders, and depression.

Differentiating TS from Other Tic Disorders

TS is one of several tic disorders, and differentiating it from other conditions is important. Key distinctions for TS include

1. **Chronic Presence of Tics** TS is characterized by both motor and vocal tics that have been present for at least one year. Other tic disorders may involve tics for shorter durations.

2. **Onset Before 18** TS typically begins in childhood, and the onset must occur before the age of 1 Other tic disorders may have different age criteria for onset.

3. **Complex Presentation** TS can include a variety of motor and vocal tics, and it is common for individuals to have a mix of simple and complex tics. In contrast, other tic disorders may involve simpler or more restricted tics.

4. **Premonitory Urge** The experience of premonitory urges, the uncomfortable sensations that precede tics, is a common feature in TS.

Treatment and Management with Medication

Medication can be an effective treatment option for managing TS, especially when tics are severe or significantly impact a person's daily life. Antipsychotic medications, such as haloperidol, risperidone, and aripiprazole, are commonly prescribed to reduce the severity of tics. These medications help regulate dopamine in the brain, which plays a role in the expression of tics.

However, medication should be used judiciously, considering individual needs and potential side effects. Treatment decisions should be made in consultation with a healthcare provider, who will assess the severity of tics, associated comorbidities, and the potential benefits and risks of medication. In some cases, behavioral therapies, such as Habit Reversal Training (HRT), may also be recommended to complement medication for managing TS.

Chapter 3 Treatment of Tourette Syndrome

What are the different treatment options for TS?

There are several treatment options for Tourette Syndrome (TS), and the most appropriate one will depend on the severity and location of the tics, as well as the individual's overall health and preferences. Here are some of the most common treatment options for TS

Behavioral therapy Behavioral therapy, such as habit reversal training or exposure and response prevention, can help individuals with TS manage their tics by teaching them strategies to reduce the frequency and severity of the tics.

Medications There are several medications that can be used to treat TS, including dopamine blockers, such as haloperidol, and dopamine agonists, such as ropinirole. These medications can help reduce the severity of tics, but they can have side effects, such as drowsiness, dizziness, and weight gain.

Deep brain stimulation Deep brain stimulation (DBS) is a surgical procedure that involves implanting a device that sends electrical impulses to the brain to help regulate tics. DBS is typically reserved for individuals with severe TS who have not responded to other treatments.

Botulinum toxin injections Botulinum toxin injections can be used to treat certain types of tics, such as eye blinking or neck twitching, by weakening the muscles involved in the tic.

Psychotherapy Psychotherapy, such as cognitive-behavioral therapy (CBT), can help individuals with TS manage their tics and improve their overall mental health and well-being.

Lifestyle modifications Making lifestyle modifications, such as avoiding stress, getting enough sleep, and engaging in regular exercise, can help individuals with TS manage their tics.

Alternative therapies Some people with TS may also find relief with alternative therapies such as meditation, yoga, or acupuncture.

It's important to note that each person with TS is unique, and what works best for one person may not work for another. A healthcare professional can work with the individual to determine the best treatment plan for their specific needs.

Deep brain stimulation (DBS) is a surgical procedure that has been shown to be effective in managing symptoms of Tourette Syndrome (TS). However, like any surgical procedure, it carries potential risks and side effects. Some of the potential side effects of DBS for TS include

Bleeding or hemorrhage There is a risk of bleeding or hemorrhage during the surgical procedure, which can lead to serious complications.

Infection As with any surgical procedure, there is a risk of infection with DBS.

Brain damage DBS involves implanting an electrode in the brain, which can cause damage to surrounding brain tissue.

Side effects from stimulation DBS can cause side effects such as numbness, weakness, or tingling in the face or limbs.

Seizures DBS can cause seizures in some individuals, particularly those with a history of seizure disorders.

Battery depletion The battery used to power the DBS device can deplete over time, which can lead to a decrease in the effectiveness of the treatment.

Technical difficulties DBS devices can malfunction or experience technical difficulties, which can lead to a decrease in the effectiveness of the treatment.

It is important to note that these side effects are not universal and may not occur in everyone who undergoes DBS for TS. It is also important to weigh the potential benefits of DBS against the potential risks and side effects.

Behavioral therapy can be used in combination with medication for TS. In fact, behavioral therapy is often used in conjunction with medication to maximize the effectiveness of treatment. Behavioral therapy can help individuals with TS to better manage their tics and improve their overall quality of life. Some common forms of behavioral therapy used to treat TS include

Habit reversal training This type of therapy helps individuals to identify and replace their tics with alternative behaviors.

Exposure and response prevention This type of therapy helps individuals to confront their tics and learn to manage them in a more effective way.

Relaxation techniques Techniques such as deep breathing, progressive muscle relaxation, and visualization can help individuals to manage their tics and reduce stress.

Lifestyle modifications that have been found to be effective for managing tics in TS include

Stress management Stress can exacerbate tics, so finding ways to manage stress, such as through relaxation techniques or exercise, can be helpful.

Avoiding stimulants Stimulants such as caffeine and nicotine can exacerbate tics, so avoiding these substances or reducing their use can be helpful.

Getting enough sleep Lack of sleep can exacerbate tics, so getting enough sleep is important.

Exercise Regular exercise has been shown to reduce tics in some individuals with TS.

Avoiding triggers Identifying and avoiding triggers for tics, such as certain environments or situations, can be helpful.

It is important to note that what works best for one individual with TS may not work for another, so it is often necessary to try

What is the role of medication in the treatment of TS?

Medication plays a significant role in the treatment of Tourette Syndrome (TS), particularly when tics are severe or significantly impair an individual's daily functioning. The primary goal of medication in TS management is to reduce the frequency and severity of tics and alleviate the distress they may cause. Here is an overview of the role of medication in TS treatment

1. **Tic Reduction** The most immediate and direct benefit of medication is the reduction of tics. Antipsychotic medications, including haloperidol, risperidone, aripiprazole, and others, are commonly prescribed for this purpose. These medications primarily work by modulating dopamine activity in the brain, which is thought to be involved in the expression of tics.

2. **Symptom Control** Medication can help individuals gain better control over their tics, allowing them to reduce their severity and frequency. This, in turn, can lead to improved quality of life and social functioning.

3. **Relief from Premonitory Urges** Some individuals with TS experience premonitory urges, which are uncomfortable sensations or feelings that precede tics. Medication can help alleviate these urges and provide relief from the distress they may cause.

4. **Reduced Social Impairment** By reducing the intensity and frequency of tics, medication can help minimize social impairment and improve an individual's ability to function in social and academic or work settings.

5. **Management of Comorbid Conditions** Many individuals with TS also experience comorbid conditions, such as Attention-Deficit/Hyperactivity Disorder (ADHD) and Obsessive-Compulsive Disorder (OCD). Medication can be used to manage these co-occurring symptoms.

6. **Enhanced Quality of Life** The overall aim of medication in TS treatment is to enhance the quality of life for individuals affected by this condition. By reducing tics and associated symptoms, medication can help individuals engage more fully in daily activities, work, school, and social interactions.

It's important to note that medication should be used judiciously, and the decision to prescribe medication should be made in consultation with a healthcare provider. Several factors, including the severity of tics, the presence of comorbid conditions, potential side effects, and individual preferences, should be considered when determining the appropriateness of medication.

Furthermore, medication is often used in conjunction with other treatment modalities, such as behavioral therapy and support from mental health professionals, to provide a comprehensive approach to TS management. The goal is to tailor treatment to the specific needs and circumstances of each individual with TS.

Potential Side Effects of Antipsychotic Medications Commonly

Prescribed for Tic Reduction in TS

Antipsychotic medications are often prescribed to reduce tics in Tourette Syndrome (TS). While they can be effective, these medications may also lead to side effects. It's important to note that not everyone will experience these side effects, and the severity can vary from person to person. Common potential side effects of antipsychotic medications for TS include

1. **Sedation** Some individuals may experience drowsiness or sedation, especially when they first start taking the medication. This effect can vary based on the specific medication.

2. **Weight Gain** Weight gain is a possible side effect, and some antipsychotic medications are associated with a higher risk of this side effect. Maintaining a balanced diet and regular physical activity can help mitigate this.

3. **Extrapyramidal Symptoms (EPS)** EPS can include symptoms like restlessness (akathisia), muscle stiffness (rigidity), and involuntary movements (dyskinesias). These symptoms are more common with first-generation antipsychotic medications.

4. **Metabolic Changes** Some antipsychotics can lead to metabolic changes, including increased blood sugar levels and lipid abnormalities. Regular monitoring of these parameters may be necessary.

5. **Prolactin Elevation** Certain antipsychotics can lead to elevated levels of the hormone prolactin, which may result in sexual dysfunction, breast enlargement (gynecomastia), and menstrual irregularities.

6. **Neuroleptic Malignant Syndrome (NMS)** While rare, NMS is a potentially life-threatening reaction to antipsychotic medications, characterized by fever, altered mental status, muscle rigidity, and autonomic dysfunction.

7. **Tardive Dyskinesia (TD)** TD is an involuntary movement disorder that can develop with long-term use of antipsychotics, particularly with first-generation antipsychotics. It is characterized by repetitive, purposeless movements.

8. **Cardiac Effects** Some antipsychotics may lead to changes in heart rate and rhythm, which may require monitoring.

It's important for individuals with TS to work closely with their healthcare provider to monitor and manage potential side effects. Medication selection should be based on the individual's specific needs, preferences, and medical history.

Behavioral Therapy Options for TS Management in Conjunction with Medication

Behavioral therapy can be used in combination with medication to enhance the management of tics in Tourette Syndrome. Some common behavioral therapy options for TS include

1. **Habit Reversal Training (HRT)** HRT is a structured, evidence-based behavioral therapy designed to increase awareness of tics and help individuals develop strategies to manage and reduce them. It includes components like identifying premonitory urges and developing competing responses.

2. **Comprehensive Behavioral Intervention for Tics (CBIT)** CBIT is a modified form of HRT that incorporates additional strategies, such as relaxation training and functional interventions. CBIT aims to help individuals understand the environmental and psychological factors that influence their tics.

3. **Exposure and Response Prevention (ERP)** ERP is typically used to manage comorbid conditions like Obsessive-Compulsive Disorder (OCD). It involves exposing individuals to obsessions (distressing thoughts) and preventing them from engaging in compulsive behaviors.

4. **Psychoeducation** Education about TS and its symptoms is essential for individuals and their families. Understanding the condition can help reduce stigma and enhance coping skills.

5. **Coping Strategies** Therapists may teach individuals with TS various coping strategies, including stress reduction techniques, relaxation exercises, and strategies for managing premonitory urges.

Determining the Most Appropriate Medication for TS

The choice of medication for Tourette Syndrome should be based on a thorough assessment by a healthcare provider. To determine the most appropriate medication, individuals with TS should consider the following factors

1. **Severity of Tics** The severity of tics and the degree to which they impair daily functioning play a significant role in medication selection.

2. **Presence of Comorbid Conditions** If an individual has co-occurring conditions like ADHD or OCD, medication choices may be influenced by their impact on these conditions as well.

3. **Potential Side Effects** Individual preferences and tolerance for potential side effects should be considered.

4. **Medical History** A person's medical history, including allergies, past responses to medications, and any existing medical conditions, will inform medication decisions.

5. **Medication Efficacy** The available research and clinical evidence regarding the effectiveness of specific medications for TS are also essential factors in decision-making.

6. **Patient Preferences** An individual's preferences and comfort with taking medication, as well as their participation in shared decision-making, are important.

Ultimately, the decision should be made collaboratively between the individual, their family (if applicable), and a qualified healthcare provider who specializes in TS management. Regular monitoring and adjustment of medication may be necessary to achieve the best outcomes.

What are the non-pharmacological treatment options for TS?

There are several non-pharmacological treatment options for Tourette Syndrome (TS), which can be used alone or in combination with medication. Some of these options include

Behavioral therapy This type of therapy helps individuals with TS to identify and change negative thought patterns and behaviors that may be contributing to their tics.

Habit reversal training This type of therapy helps individuals with TS to identify and replace their tics with alternative behaviors.

Exposure and response prevention This type of therapy helps individuals with TS to confront their tics and learn to manage them in a more effective way.

Cognitive-behavioral therapy This type of therapy helps individuals with TS to identify and change negative thought patterns and behaviors that may be contributing to their tics.

Psychodynamic therapy This type of therapy helps individuals with TS to understand and resolve any underlying psychological conflicts that may be contributing to their tics.

Speech therapy This type of therapy helps individuals with TS to improve their communication skills and reduce the severity of their tics.

Occupational therapy This type of therapy helps individuals with TS to develop strategies to manage their tics and improve their ability to function in daily life.

Physical therapy This type of therapy helps individuals with TS to improve their physical functioning and reduce the severity of their tics.

Mindfulness meditation This type of therapy helps individuals with TS to become more aware of their thoughts and feelings and to manage their tics in a more effective way.

Biofeedback This type of therapy helps individuals with TS to become more aware of their body's physiological responses and to learn to control their tics.

Neurofeedback This type of therapy helps individuals with TS to become more aware of their brain's activity and to learn to control their tics.

Relaxation techniques Techniques such as deep breathing, progressive muscle relaxation, and visualization can help individuals with TS to manage their tics and reduce stress.

Sensory integration therapy This type of therapy helps individuals with TS to process and integrate sensory information more effectively, which can help to reduce tics.

Animal-assisted therapy This type of therapy uses animals, such as dogs, to help individuals with TS to manage their tics and improve their social and emotional functioning.

Music therapy This type of therapy uses music to help individuals with TS to manage their tics and improve their mood and social functioning.

Art therapy This type of therapy uses art-making to help individuals with TS to express and process their emotions and to manage their tics.

Drama therapy This type of therapy uses drama and acting techniques to help individuals with TS to manage their tics and improve their social and emotional functioning.

Yoga and tai chi These mind-body practices can help individuals with TS to manage their tics and improve their overall well-being.

Massage therapy Massage can help individuals with TS to relax and reduce muscle tension, which can help to manage tics.

Acupuncture This traditional Chinese medicine technique involves the insertion of thin needles into specific points on the body to help manage tics and improve overall well-being.

It's important to note that each individual with TS is unique, and what works best for one person may not work for another. A healthcare professional can help determine the most appropriate non-pharmacological treatment options for each individual.

Habit Reversal Training (HRT) for TS

Habit Reversal Training (HRT) is a well-established and effective behavioral therapy used in the management of tics in Tourette Syndrome (TS). HRT is based on the premise that tics are learned behaviors and that individuals can gain control over them through awareness and self-regulation. Here's how HRT typically works

1. **Awareness Training** The first step of HRT is to help individuals with TS become more aware of their tics. This involves identifying when tics are about to occur or when they experience premonitory urges, which are uncomfortable sensations that precede tics. Developing this awareness is crucial because it provides a foundation for control.

2. **Competing Response** In HRT, individuals are taught to develop a specific, voluntary response that is physically incompatible with their tics. For example, if someone has a motor tic that involves raising their shoulder, the competing response might be to contract the

shoulder muscle on the opposite side. The competing response serves to interrupt the tic and reduce its occurrence.

3. **Premonitory Urge Awareness** HRT also helps individuals recognize the premonitory urges that precede tics. Learning to identify these urges can provide an early warning system for tics and help individuals respond with a competing behavior.

4. **Contingency Management** Contingency management is used to reinforce the use of competing responses. Individuals receive positive feedback and rewards for successfully implementing the competing response, which encourages its consistent use.

5. **Social Support** A supportive and understanding social environment is essential for the success of HRT. Family and friends play a critical role in providing encouragement and assistance.

HRT is typically delivered by a trained therapist, and it involves regular sessions and homework assignments to practice the learned techniques. The skills acquired in HRT can help individuals with TS reduce the frequency and severity of their tics and gain better control over their symptoms.

Exposure and Response Prevention (ERP) Therapy for TS

Exposure and Response Prevention (ERP) therapy is a form of cognitive-behavioral therapy (CBT) often used to manage comorbid conditions like Obsessive-Compulsive Disorder (OCD), which frequently co-occurs with Tourette Syndrome (TS). In the context of TS, ERP can help individuals manage their tics and related premonitory urges by applying the following principles

1. **Exposure** Individuals are gradually exposed to situations or stimuli that trigger their obsessive thoughts and tics. Exposure is done in a controlled and systematic manner.

2. **Response Prevention** During exposure, individuals are prevented from engaging in their typical compulsive behaviors or tics. This process helps break the cycle of obsessions and compulsions.

3. **Functional Assessment** Therapists work with individuals to identify the environmental and psychological triggers for tics and obsessive thoughts. Understanding these triggers can guide the development of exposure exercises.

4. **Homework and Practice** Individuals are often encouraged to practice exposure exercises outside of therapy sessions to generalize the skills they've learned. This helps them confront their triggers and practice not engaging in the tic response.

ERP can be effective in helping individuals with TS reduce the impact of tics and premonitory urges. It provides a structured and evidence-based approach to symptom management and is particularly useful for individuals with co-occurring OCD.

Occupational Therapy Strategies for TS

Occupational therapy can be a valuable part of a comprehensive treatment plan for individuals with Tourette Syndrome. Occupational therapists can help individuals develop strategies to manage their tics and associated challenges. Some strategies that may be used in occupational therapy for TS include

1. **Sensory Integration Techniques** Occupational therapists may employ sensory integration strategies to help individuals manage sensory sensitivities that can trigger tics. Sensory integration techniques aim to desensitize individuals to sensory stimuli gradually.

2. **Stress Management** Occupational therapists can teach stress-reduction techniques, such as deep breathing exercises, mindfulness,

and progressive muscle relaxation, to help individuals manage anxiety and stress, which can exacerbate tics.

3. **Time Management and Organization** TS can impact an individual's ability to manage time and stay organized. Occupational therapists can provide tools and strategies to improve these skills.

4. **School and Workplace Accommodations** Occupational therapists can help individuals with TS access accommodations at school or work to support their needs, such as extended time for tasks or modifications to their environment.

5. **Social Skills Training** Occupational therapy can include social skills training to help individuals with TS navigate social interactions and improve their self-esteem.

6. **Fine Motor Skills Development** For individuals with TS that experience motor tics, occupational therapists can work on fine motor skills to help with tasks like handwriting and other fine motor activities.

Occupational therapy is highly individualized, and the specific strategies and interventions will vary depending on the needs and goals of the person with TS. Occupational therapists collaborate with individuals and their families to develop a tailored plan for addressing the challenges associated with TS.

Chapter 4

Impact of Tourette Syndrome on Daily Life

How does TS affect school performance?

Tourette Syndrome (TS) can have a significant impact on an individual's school performance, as it can affect their ability to concentrate, learn, and interact with their peers. Here are some ways in which TS can affect school performance

Difficulty with attention and concentration TS can cause individuals to have difficulty paying attention and concentrating, which can affect their ability to learn and retain information.

Impulsivity TS can cause individuals to have difficulty controlling their impulses, which can lead to disruptive behavior in the classroom, such as interrupting the teacher or blurting out answers.

Memory and learning difficulties TS can affect an individual's short-term and working memory, making it difficult for them to learn and remember new information.

Social difficulties TS can cause individuals to have difficulty interacting with their peers, which can lead to social isolation and difficulties with teamwork and collaboration.

Emotional difficulties TS can cause individuals to experience anxiety, depression, and other emotional difficulties, which can affect their ability to perform well in school.

Sensory sensitivities TS can cause individuals to be oversensitive to certain sounds, sights, or other sensory stimuli, which can be distracting and affect their ability to focus in the classroom.

Motor tics TS can cause individuals to have motor tics, such as eye blinking, head jerking, or hand flapping, which can be distracting and affect their ability to perform tasks that require fine motor skills.

Vocal tics TS can cause individuals to have vocal tics, such as grunting, sniffing, or clearing their throat, which can be disruptive and affect their ability to communicate effectively.

Stigma and bullying TS can be stigmatized, and individuals with TS may be subject to bullying and teasing, which can affect their self-esteem and ability to perform well in school.

It's important to note that every individual with TS is different, and the impact of TS on school performance can vary widely. Some individuals with TS may experience few or no difficulties, while others may face significant challenges. It's important for teachers, counselors, and other educational professionals to be aware of the effects of TS and to provide appropriate accommodations and support to help individuals with TS succeed in school.

Strategies for Teachers to Support Students with TS in the Classroom

Supporting students with Tourette Syndrome (TS) in the classroom requires understanding, patience, and flexibility. Here are some strategies that teachers can use to create a supportive learning environment

1. **Education and Awareness** Educate yourself and your students about TS to reduce stigma and promote understanding. Discuss TS with the class and emphasize that it is a neurological condition beyond the student's control.

2. **Communication** Maintain open lines of communication with the student, their parents, and any special education professionals involved in their care. Regularly check in to see how the student is feeling and whether they need any accommodations or adjustments.

3. **Flexible Seating** Allow the student to choose a seat that is least distracting for them. This might mean sitting near the front, away from potential triggers, or in a quieter part of the classroom.

4. **Frequent Breaks** Recognize that students with TS may benefit from brief breaks to help manage tics and premonitory urges. These breaks can be structured into the daily schedule.

5. **Extended Time for Tasks** Offer extended time for assignments and tests if the student requires it due to tic-related interruptions.

6. **Alternative Assessments** Provide alternatives to written assessments, such as oral presentations, video projects, or digital assignments, to accommodate students with writing or fine motor tics.

7. **Quiet Space** Create a designated quiet area in the classroom where the student can retreat if needed.

8. **Use of Technology** Encourage the use of assistive technology, such as voice-to-text software or digital notes, to assist with written tasks.

9. **Positive Reinforcement** Recognize and reward the student's efforts and achievements, which can boost their self-esteem.

10. **Support Peer Understanding** Educate the student's peers about TS and foster a supportive and inclusive classroom community.

Accommodations and Resources to Support Students with TS

Students with TS may benefit from various accommodations and resources to help them succeed in school. Some of these include

1. **Individualized Education Plan (IEP) or 504 Plan** These legal documents can outline specific accommodations and supports for students with TS. They may include extended time on tests, breaks, or access to assistive technology.

2. **School Counselors** School counselors can provide emotional support and help students develop strategies to cope with stress and anxiety related to TS.

3. **Occupational Therapy** Some students with TS may benefit from occupational therapy to improve fine motor skills and manage sensory sensitivities.

4. **Speech Therapy** Speech therapy can be helpful for students with vocal tics or communication difficulties.

5. **Supportive Teaching Assistants** Having a teaching assistant in the classroom can provide extra support and ensure that accommodations are implemented effectively.

6. **Quiet Spaces** Designated quiet spaces can be created within the school where students can take breaks if their tics become overwhelming.

7. **Access to Educational Technology** Providing access to technology can help students with TS overcome challenges related to writing or fine motor tics.

8. **Support Groups** Encourage participation in support groups for students with TS, where they can share experiences and strategies for managing their condition.

Support from Parents and Caregivers

Parents and caregivers play a crucial role in supporting their child with TS in their academic journey. Here are some ways they can provide support

1. **Communication** Maintain open and regular communication with teachers, school staff, and support professionals to ensure that the child's needs are met.

2. **Advocate for Accommodations** Work with the school to establish an IEP or 504 Plan that outlines necessary accommodations and supports.

3. **Educational Support** Help with homework and provide additional educational support as needed. Create a quiet and organized study space at home.

4. **Emotional Support** Offer emotional support and encouragement. Acknowledge your child's efforts and successes.

5. **Self-Advocacy Skills** Encourage your child to develop self-advocacy skills, including expressing their needs to teachers and peers.

6. **Stress Management** Teach stress-management techniques and provide a calming environment at home.

7. **Supportive Environment** Foster a supportive and understanding home environment to reduce stress and anxiety.

8. **Access Resources** Connect with TS support organizations and resources to gain knowledge and access additional support.

By working together with educators and support professionals, parents and caregivers can help their child with TS succeed in school and navigate the challenges associated with their condition.

How does TS affect social interactions?

Tourette Syndrome (TS) can significantly affect an individual's social interactions, as it can impact their ability to communicate and interact with others. Here are some ways in which TS can affect social interactions

Stuttering or vocal tics Individuals with TS may experience stuttering or vocal tics, such as grunting, sniffing, or clearing their throat, which can make it difficult for them to communicate effectively. This can lead to anxiety and self-consciousness in social situations.

Social anxiety The stigma surrounding TS can lead to social anxiety, as individuals with TS may feel embarrassed or ashamed of their condition. This can cause them to avoid social situations or feel uncomfortable in new environments.

Difficulty with eye contact Individuals with TS may have difficulty maintaining eye contact, which can be misinterpreted as a lack of interest or engagement. This can make it difficult to build relationships or communicate effectively.

Misunderstandings TS can cause individuals to have difficulty with impulse control, leading to sudden movements or outbursts. This can be misinterpreted as aggressive or disruptive behavior, leading to social misunderstandings and conflicts.

Social isolation The challenges associated with TS can lead to social isolation, as individuals with TS may avoid social situations or feel uncomfortable in new environments. This can lead to feelings of loneliness and depression.

Difficulty with initiating or sustaining conversations Individuals with TS may have difficulty initiating or sustaining conversations, as they may experience anxiety or difficulty with word-finding. This can make it challenging to build relationships or engage in social interactions.

Difficulty with understanding social cues Individuals with TS may have difficulty understanding social cues, such as facial expressions or body language. This can lead to difficulties in interpreting social situations or responding appropriately.

Sensory sensitivities TS can cause individuals to be oversensitive to certain sounds, sights, or other sensory stimuli. This can make it challenging to navigate social situations, such as loud restaurants or crowded spaces.

It's important to note that every individual with TS is different, and the impact of TS on social interactions can vary widely. Some individuals with TS may experience few or no difficulties, while others may face significant challenges. It's important for individuals with TS to seek support from healthcare professionals, family, and friends to help them navigate social interactions and build fulfilling relationships.

Strategies for Improving Social Interactions in Individuals with TS

Improving social interactions for individuals with Tourette Syndrome (TS) involves developing self-awareness, self-advocacy, and effective communication skills. Here are some strategies and techniques that can help

1. **Self-Awareness** Encourage individuals with TS to understand their condition, including their tics and premonitory urges. Knowing their triggers and patterns can help them anticipate and manage their symptoms.

2. **Self-Advocacy** Teach individuals with TS to communicate their needs to others, including friends, family, and teachers. Encourage them to express when they need accommodations or understanding.

3. **Practice Coping Strategies** Help individuals develop strategies to manage stress and anxiety, as these can exacerbate tics and impact social interactions. Deep breathing, mindfulness, and relaxation techniques can be beneficial.

4. **Educate Peers** Encourage the individual to educate their friends and peers about TS. Explain that tics are involuntary and uncontrollable movements or sounds. Reducing stigma and increasing understanding can lead to more supportive social interactions.

5. **Preparation** Prepare individuals with TS for social situations by discussing potential challenges and strategies for managing their tics. This can boost their confidence and reduce anxiety.

6. **Positive Self-Talk** Promote a positive self-image and self-esteem. Individuals with TS should focus on their strengths and capabilities rather than their condition.

7. **Join Support Groups** Encourage participation in TS support groups, where they can connect with others facing similar challenges, share experiences, and exchange coping strategies.

Support Groups and Resources for Individuals with TS

There are several support groups and resources available to help individuals with TS connect with others and access valuable information and support

1. **Tourette Association of America** This national organization offers resources, support, and information for individuals and families affected by TS. They provide online forums, webinars, and local support groups.

2. **Local TS Support Groups** Many regions have local TS support groups that offer in-person meetings and opportunities to connect with others in the community.

3. **Online Communities** Various online communities and forums, such as social media groups and Reddit's r/Tourettes, provide a platform for individuals to share experiences and receive support.

4. **Therapy and Counseling** Mental health professionals, such as psychologists and social workers, can provide therapy and support tailored to individuals with TS and their specific social challenges.

How Friends and Family Can Best Support Individuals with TS in Their Social Interactions

Support from friends and family is invaluable in helping individuals with TS navigate social interactions. Here are some ways to provide effective support

1. **Listen and Be Empathetic** Be a good listener and show empathy. Let the individual express their feelings and experiences without judgment.

2. **Educate Yourself** Learn about TS, its symptoms, and its impact on social interactions. This knowledge will help you better understand the challenges the individual faces.

3. **Encourage Self-Advocacy** Encourage the person with TS to communicate their needs and preferences. Offer your assistance in advocating for accommodations when necessary.

4. **Reduce Stigma** Educate others about TS and promote understanding. Correct misconceptions and stereotypes when they arise.

5. **Respect Privacy** Respect the individual's privacy and boundaries. Do not pressure them to discuss their condition if they are not comfortable doing so.

6. **Provide Emotional Support** Offer emotional support during challenging social situations. Help the individual build resilience and cope with anxiety.

7. **Participate in Supportive Activities** Engage in activities that the individual enjoys and feels comfortable with. Supportive hobbies and interests can help strengthen social connections.

8. **Create an Inclusive Environment** Foster a welcoming and inclusive environment at home and in social settings. Encourage positive interactions and understanding among family members and friends.

9. **Connect with Support Resources** Seek out local or online support groups and resources to connect with others who can provide guidance and share experiences.

By offering understanding, empathy, and encouragement, friends and family can play a vital role in helping individuals with TS feel supported and confident in their social interactions.

How does TS affect mental health?

Tourette Syndrome (TS) can have a significant impact on an individual's mental health and well-being. The condition can affect a person's self-esteem, self-confidence, and overall quality of life. Here are some ways in which TS can affect mental health

Anxiety TS can cause individuals to experience anxiety, especially in social situations. They may feel self-conscious about their tics and worry about being judged or stigmatized.

Depression Individuals with TS may experience depression, which can be related to the challenges of living with the condition. They may feel frustrated, isolated, and hopeless.

Emotional regulation TS can affect an individual's ability to regulate their emotions. They may experience mood swings, irritability, and difficulty managing stress.

Social isolation TS can make it difficult for individuals to participate in social activities and maintain relationships. They may feel embarrassed or ashamed of their tics, leading to social isolation and loneliness.

Stigma The stigma surrounding TS can lead to feelings of shame, embarrassment, and low self-esteem. Individuals with TS may feel like they are "different" or "abnormal."

Cognitive distortions TS can affect an individual's cognitive functioning, leading to cognitive distortions such as negative self-talk, all-or-nothing thinking, and overgeneralization.

Sleep disturbances TS can affect sleep patterns, leading to insomnia, daytime fatigue, and other sleep-related problems.

Anger and aggression TS can cause individuals to experience anger and aggression, which can be directed towards themselves or others.

Obsessive-compulsive behavior TS can lead to obsessive-compulsive behavior, such as repetitive thoughts or actions.

Suicidal ideation In severe cases, TS can lead to suicidal ideation and attempts. It's essential to seek professional help if such thoughts occur.

It's important to note that not everyone with TS will experience these mental health challenges, and the severity of the condition can vary widely. However, it's crucial to be aware of the potential impact of TS on mental health and seek professional help if needed. With appropriate treatment and support, individuals with TS can lead fulfilling lives and manage their mental health effectively.

Effective Treatments for Managing Mental Health Challenges Associated with TS

Individuals with Tourette Syndrome (TS) may experience various mental health challenges, including anxiety, depression, and obsessive-compulsive symptoms. Effective treatments for managing these challenges can include

1. **Cognitive-Behavioral Therapy (CBT)** CBT is a well-established approach for addressing anxiety and mood disorders. It helps individuals identify and change negative thought patterns, develop coping strategies, and manage anxiety and depression.

2. **Exposure and Response Prevention (ERP)** ERP is used to address obsessive-compulsive symptoms often seen in individuals with TS. It involves exposing individuals to distressing thoughts and preventing them from engaging in compulsive behaviors.

3. **Medication** In some cases, medication may be prescribed to manage anxiety, depression, or obsessive-compulsive symptoms. Selective serotonin reuptake inhibitors (SSRIs) are commonly used for these purposes.

4. **Supportive Psychotherapy** Supportive psychotherapy provides a safe and empathetic space for individuals to discuss their concerns and emotions. It can help alleviate emotional distress associated with TS.

5. **Mindfulness and Relaxation Techniques** Mindfulness practices and relaxation techniques can be helpful in reducing stress and improving emotional well-being.

6. **Social Support** Building a strong social support network can provide emotional assistance and reduce feelings of isolation.

7. **Psychoeducation** Learning more about TS, its symptoms, and its impact on mental health can be empowering. It helps individuals and their families better understand and cope with the condition.

Support Groups and Resources for Individuals with TS and Their Families

Several support groups and resources are available for individuals with TS and their families

1. **Tourette Association of America** This national organization offers a range of resources, including information on TS, support groups, webinars, and educational materials.

2. **Local TS Support Groups** Many regions have local support groups that hold meetings and events where individuals and families can connect with others in their community.

3. **Online Communities** Online forums and social media groups dedicated to TS provide platforms for sharing experiences, seeking advice, and finding support.

4. **Mental Health Professionals** Consult with mental health professionals who specialize in TS or related conditions for tailored support.

5. **Family and Friends** Engage your immediate social network for emotional support. Loved ones can be a valuable source of understanding and assistance.

6. **School Resources** Schools may have counselors or special education staff who can provide support and accommodations for students with TS.

7. **Mental Health Hotlines** Crisis hotlines, such as the National Suicide Prevention Lifeline, are available for individuals experiencing severe emotional distress.

Impact of TS on Cognitive Functioning and Cognitive Distortions

Tourette Syndrome (TS) can have some impact on cognitive functioning, primarily due to the presence of tics and associated mental processes. These effects are not universal and can vary from person to person. Common cognitive effects include

1. **Cognitive Load** Tics, especially when frequent or severe, can increase cognitive load, making it more challenging for individuals to concentrate and process information.

2. **Premonitory Urges** Premonitory urges, which precede tics, can consume cognitive resources and lead to cognitive distraction or a sense of discomfort.

3. **Cognitive Flexibility** Some individuals with TS may experience difficulties with cognitive flexibility, such as shifting between tasks or adapting to changes in routines.

Cognitive distortions, on the other hand, are thought patterns that contribute to negative emotions and behaviors. While they are not directly caused by TS, individuals with TS, especially those who experience comorbid conditions like anxiety, may develop cognitive distortions related to their tics, premonitory urges, or social interactions. These distortions can include

1. **Catastrophizing** Believing that tics or their consequences are much worse than they actually are.

2. **Mind Reading** Assuming that others are constantly judging or negatively evaluating their tics.

3. **Personalization** Believing that their tics or behaviors are responsible for external events or other people's reactions.

Cognitive-behavioral therapy (CBT) is a valuable approach for addressing cognitive distortions and helping individuals reframe their thought patterns to reduce emotional distress and improve mental well-being. It can be particularly useful for individuals with TS who are dealing with anxiety and depression related to their condition.

Chapter 5

Comorbidity with Tourette Syndrome

What are the most common comorbidities of TS?

Tourette Syndrome (TS) is a neurodevelopmental disorder characterized by motor and vocal tics, and it can often co-occur with other conditions or comorbidities. Some of the most common comorbidities of TS include

Attention Deficit Hyperactivity Disorder (ADHD) ADHD is a common comorbidity of TS, and it is estimated that up to 70% of individuals with TS also have ADHD.

Obsessive-Compulsive Disorder (OCD) OCD is another common comorbidity of TS, and it is estimated that up to 50% of individuals with TS also have OCD.

Anxiety Disorders Anxiety disorders, such as generalized anxiety disorder, social anxiety disorder, and panic disorder, are common in individuals with TS.

Depression Depression is a common comorbidity of TS, and it is estimated that up to 50% of individuals with TS will experience depression at some point in their lives.

Sleep Disorders Sleep disorders, such as insomnia, sleep apnea, and restless leg syndrome, are common in individuals with TS.

Learning Disabilities Learning disabilities, such as dyslexia, dyscalculia, and dysgraphia, are common in individuals with TS.

Speech and Language Disorders Speech and language disorders, such as stuttering, articulation difficulties, and language processing difficulties, are common in individuals with TS.

Social Skills Deficits Individuals with TS may experience social skills deficits, such as difficulty with eye contact, initiating and maintaining conversations, and understanding social cues.

Executive Function Deficits Executive function deficits, such as difficulty with planning, organization, and time management, are common in individuals with TS.

Tic-Related Disorders Tic-related disorders, such as coprolalia (the urge to utter obscene words or phrases) and echolalia (the repetition of words or phrases), can also occur in individuals with TS.

It is important to note that the severity and frequency of these comorbidities can vary widely from person to person, and not all individuals with TS will experience all of them. However, it is important to be aware of these common comorbidities and to seek professional help if symptoms persist or worsen over time.

Treatment Options for Individuals with TS and Comorbidities

Individuals with Tourette Syndrome (TS) often experience comorbid conditions, such as Attention-Deficit/Hyperactivity Disorder (ADHD), Obsessive-Compulsive Disorder (OCD), anxiety, and mood disorders. Effective treatment for individuals with TS and comorbidities typically involves a combination of approaches

1. **Medication** Depending on the specific comorbidity, medication may be prescribed. For ADHD, stimulants like methylphenidate or non-stimulant medications may be used. Selective serotonin reuptake inhibitors (SSRIs) are often prescribed for OCD and anxiety.

2. **Behavioral Therapy** Behavioral therapies, such as Cognitive-Behavioral Therapy (CBT) or Exposure and Response Prevention (ERP), can be used to address comorbid conditions like OCD and anxiety.

3. **Habit Reversal Training (HRT)** HRT, a behavioral therapy, can help individuals manage tics and related comorbid conditions, such as OCD.

4. **Supportive Psychotherapy** Supportive psychotherapy provides a safe and empathetic space for individuals to discuss their experiences and emotions, which can be particularly helpful for mood disorders.

5. **Psychoeducation** Learning more about the comorbid conditions and their treatment options can be empowering for individuals and their families.

6. **Lifestyle Management** Adopting a healthy lifestyle that includes regular exercise, a balanced diet, and stress-reduction techniques can complement other treatments.

7. **Support Groups** Joining support groups that focus on specific comorbidities, such as ADHD or OCD, can provide a platform for individuals to connect with others and share experiences and strategies.

Relationship Between TS and Tic-Related Disorders

Tic-related disorders are conditions characterized by the presence of tics but without meeting the full criteria for TS. These disorders include

1. **Persistent (Chronic) Motor or Vocal Tic Disorder** Individuals with this disorder experience either motor or vocal tics, but not both, for more than a year. The tics may be present daily or intermittently.

2. **Provisional Tic Disorder** Provisional tic disorder is diagnosed in children who have tics that have been present for less than a year. It often precedes a diagnosis of TS.

3. **Tourettism** Tourettism refers to tics that occur in the context of another neurological or medical condition, such as autism or Huntington's disease.

While these disorders share some characteristics with TS, they differ in terms of the duration, complexity, and presence of both motor and vocal tics. Individuals with tic-related disorders may experience tics that are less frequent or less complex than those seen in TS. However, these conditions

83

can still impact daily life and may benefit from treatment, particularly if they are associated with distress or functional impairment.

Support Groups and Resources for Individuals with TS and Comorbidities

Support groups and resources are available for individuals with TS and their families who are dealing with comorbidities

1. **Tourette Association of America** This national organization provides resources, support groups, and educational materials for individuals and families dealing with TS and its comorbidities.

2. **Local Support Groups** Many regions have local TS support groups that offer meetings and resources to help individuals and families connect with others facing similar challenges.

3. **Online Communities** Various online communities and forums dedicated to TS and related conditions can be sources of information, advice, and support.

4. **Mental Health Organizations** Organizations dedicated to specific comorbid conditions, such as the Anxiety and Depression Association of America (ADAA) or Children and Adults with Attention-Deficit/Hyperactivity Disorder (CHADD), provide information and resources.

By accessing these support groups and resources, individuals and families can find guidance, connect with others, and gain valuable information to help them manage both TS and its comorbidities.

How are comorbidities treated in patients with TS?

Treating comorbidities in patients with Tourette Syndrome (TS) can be challenging, as it requires a comprehensive approach that addresses both the tics and the comorbid condition. The treatment approach may vary depending on the specific comorbidity and its severity, as well as the individual patient's needs and response to therapy. Here are some common approaches to treating comorbidities in patients with TS

Medications Medications may be prescribed to treat both tics and comorbid conditions. For example, dopamine blockers such as haloperidol or pimozide can help reduce tics, while antipsychotic medications such as risperidone or aripiprazole can help manage associated behaviors such as aggression or impulsivity. Antidepressants may also be prescribed to treat comorbid conditions such as obsessive-compulsive disorder (OCD) or anxiety disorders.

Behavioral therapy Behavioral therapy, such as cognitive-behavioral therapy (CBT), can be effective in managing comorbid conditions such as OCD or anxiety disorders. CBT can help patients identify and change negative thought patterns and behaviors that contribute to their symptoms. Exposure and response prevention (ERP) therapy, a form of CBT, can help patients confront their fears and reduce compulsive behaviors.

Habit reversal training Habit reversal training is a behavioral therapy technique that can help patients replace tics with more constructive behaviors. For example, a patient with a tic that involves blinking may learn to replace it with a different behavior, such as tapping their foot.

Tic management Tic management techniques, such as biofeedback or progressive muscle relaxation, can help patients become more aware of their tics and learn to manage them more effectively.

Psychotherapy Psychotherapy, such as individual or family therapy, can be helpful in addressing the emotional and psychological impact of TS and comorbid conditions. It can also provide support and education to patients and their families.

Lifestyle modifications Lifestyle modifications, such as regular exercise, stress management, and sleep hygiene, can help reduce tics and improve overall mental health.

Deep brain stimulation Deep brain stimulation (DBS) is a surgical procedure that involves implanting a device that delivers electrical impulses to specific areas of the brain. DBS has been shown to be effective in reducing tics in some patients with TS, and may also help manage comorbid conditions such as OCD or depression.

It's important to note that each patient with TS is unique, and the most effective treatment approach will depend on the individual patient's needs and circumstances. A healthcare professional, such as a neurologist or psychiatrist, should be consulted to determine the best course of treatment.

Common Comorbid Conditions with TS

Individuals with Tourette Syndrome (TS) often experience comorbid conditions, which can complicate their overall health and well-being. Some of the common comorbid conditions associated with TS include

1. **Attention-Deficit/Hyperactivity Disorder (ADHD)** Many individuals with TS also have ADHD, characterized by symptoms of inattention, hyperactivity, and impulsivity.

2. **Obsessive-Compulsive Disorder (OCD)** OCD involves intrusive, distressing thoughts (obsessions) and repetitive, ritualistic behaviors (compulsions). It often co-occurs with TS.

3. **Anxiety Disorders** Individuals with TS may experience various anxiety disorders, such as generalized anxiety disorder, social anxiety disorder, or specific phobias.

4. **Mood Disorders** Depression and bipolar disorder can co-occur with TS, leading to mood swings, low energy, and changes in affect.

5. **Sleep Disorders** Sleep problems, including insomnia and sleep-related movement disorders, can affect individuals with TS.

6. **Learning Disabilities** Some individuals with TS may also have learning disabilities, which can impact their educational performance.

7. **Behavioral Disorders** Oppositional defiant disorder and conduct disorder may be more common in individuals with TS, especially when associated with ADHD.

8. **Sensory Processing Disorder** Sensory sensitivities or difficulties in processing sensory information can be present in individuals with TS.

9. **Autism Spectrum Disorders (ASD)** While not a direct comorbidity, some individuals with TS may have features of ASD or co-occurring ASD.

Deep Brain Stimulation (DBS) and Its Effectiveness in Treating TS

Deep Brain Stimulation (DBS) is a neurosurgical procedure that involves implanting electrodes into specific areas of the brain to modulate abnormal neural activity. DBS has been investigated as a treatment option for severe cases of TS that do not respond to other therapies.

The effectiveness of DBS in treating TS varies among individuals. Some studies have reported significant tic reduction and improvements in overall quality of life for certain patients. However, it is crucial to understand that DBS is considered a last-resort treatment and is not appropriate for all individuals with TS. Potential benefits of DBS include

1. **Tic Reduction** DBS can lead to a significant reduction in both motor and vocal tics, which can be particularly beneficial for individuals with severe, debilitating tics.

2. **Improved Functioning** Some patients experience improved functioning in daily life, including better control over their tics and reduced interference with daily activities.

3. **Quality of Life** Many individuals report an enhanced quality of life, reduced distress, and an overall sense of well-being following successful DBS treatment.

However, it's important to be aware of the potential risks and limitations of DBS, including surgical risks, side effects, and the fact that not all patients experience the same degree of benefit. DBS is typically considered when other treatments have been unsuccessful, and it should be carefully evaluated on a case-by-case basis.

Alternative Treatments or Therapies for Managing Comorbidities in TS

While there is no one-size-fits-all alternative treatment for comorbid conditions in TS, several complementary and alternative therapies may help manage symptoms and improve overall well-being. These may include

1. **Mindfulness and Meditation** Mindfulness practices can reduce stress and anxiety associated with comorbid conditions, improving emotional well-being.

2. **Yoga** Yoga combines physical postures, breathing exercises, and meditation to enhance relaxation and reduce anxiety and depression symptoms.

3. **Nutrition and Diet** A well-balanced diet can support overall health and may benefit individuals with comorbid conditions.

4. **Exercise** Regular physical activity can help alleviate mood symptoms and improve overall mental health.

5. **Biofeedback and Relaxation Techniques** Biofeedback and relaxation therapies teach individuals to manage physiological responses to stress and anxiety.

6. **Art and Music Therapy** These therapies can provide a creative outlet for emotional expression and stress reduction.

It's essential to consult with healthcare professionals and specialists to discuss the suitability and effectiveness of alternative treatments for specific comorbid conditions. These treatments are often used as complementary strategies alongside evidence-based medical and psychological therapies.

Chapter 6

Tourette Syndrome in the Classroom

What accommodations can be made for students with TS in the classroom?

There are several accommodations that can be made for students with Tourette Syndrome (TS) in the classroom to help them learn and succeed. Here are some common accommodations

Seating arrangement Providing a quiet and comfortable seating arrangement for the student can help reduce distractions and minimize the impact of tics.

Tic-friendly environment Creating a tic-friendly environment in the classroom can help the student feel more at ease. This can include allowing the student to use a stress ball, fidget toy, or other devices that can help them manage their tics.

Adapted assignments Providing adapted assignments that take into account the student's strengths and challenges can help them complete tasks successfully. For example, allowing the student to use a computer for written assignments instead of writing by hand can help reduce the impact of motor tics.

Extra time Providing extra time for assignments, tests, and other activities can help the student manage their tics and complete tasks without feeling rushed or overwhelmed.

Use of assistive technology Assistive technology, such as text-to-speech software or a speech-to-text device, can help the student communicate more effectively and reduce the impact of tics on their schoolwork.

Classroom modifications Making modifications to the classroom environment, such as reducing noise levels or providing a private workspace, can help the student focus and manage their tics.

Support from a teaching assistant Providing a teaching assistant to support the student in the classroom can help them stay on task, manage their tics, and provide additional support as needed.

Social skills training Providing social skills training for the student can help them develop strategies for managing social interactions and reducing anxiety and stress related to tics.

Counseling Providing counseling for the student can help them develop coping strategies for managing tics and anxiety, as well as provide support and guidance for navigating social situations.

Education and awareness Educating the student's classmates and teachers about TS can help increase understanding and acceptance, reduce stigma, and create a more supportive environment for the student.

It's important to note that each student with TS is unique, and the most effective accommodations will depend on the individual student's needs and circumstances. Working closely with the student, their family, and other educational professionals can help ensure that the accommodations are tailored to meet their specific needs and help them succeed in the classroom.

Determining Effective Accommodations for Students with TS

Determining the most effective accommodations for a student with Tourette Syndrome (TS) involves collaboration between the student, their parents, teachers, and possibly special education professionals. Here's a step-by-step approach to identify appropriate accommodations

1. **Assessment** Conduct an assessment of the student's specific needs. This may involve reviewing their medical and educational history, observing their tics and their impact on learning, and considering any comorbid conditions, such as ADHD or OCD.

2. **Individualized Education Plan (IEP) or 504 Plan** If the student has been identified as eligible for special education services, work with the school to develop an IEP or a 504 Plan. These legally mandated plans outline the accommodations and supports required to meet the student's needs.

3. **Consult with Specialists** Consult with specialists, such as a school psychologist or a neuropsychologist, who can provide insights into the student's cognitive, emotional, and behavioral profile. They can help identify appropriate accommodations.

4. **Parent and Student Input** Include the student and their parents in the accommodation decision-making process. They can provide valuable input regarding the student's unique needs and preferences.

5. **Trial and Review** Implement accommodations on a trial basis to assess their effectiveness. Periodically review and adjust the accommodations as needed based on the student's progress and changing needs.

6. **Professional Development** Ensure that teachers and school staff receive professional development on TS and its accommodations. This education is critical for effective implementation.

7. **Regular Communication** Maintain open lines of communication between the student, parents, and teachers. Regularly check in to discuss the effectiveness of accommodations and make necessary adjustments.

Strategies and Resources for Social Skills Training

Effective social skills training is crucial for students with TS. Here are some strategies and resources

1. **Role-Playing** Role-playing social situations can help students practice appropriate responses to common interactions.

2. **Social Stories** Social stories are short narratives that describe specific social situations and appropriate responses. They can help students with TS better understand and navigate social scenarios.

3. **Group Activities** Encourage participation in group activities and projects that promote teamwork and social interaction. These can be part of the regular curriculum or extracurricular activities.

4. **Peer Mentoring** Pair the student with a peer mentor who can provide guidance and support in social situations.

5. **Social Skills Curriculum** Use structured social skills curricula that address specific areas of social interaction, such as conversation skills, empathy, and conflict resolution.

6. **Social Skills Apps and Games** There are several apps and games designed to teach and reinforce social skills. These can be used both in and out of the classroom.

7. **Social Skills Groups** Consider enrolling the student in social skills groups led by a trained therapist or counselor.

8. **Communication with School Counselors** School counselors can play a valuable role in providing social skills training and supporting the student's social development.

Educating Classmates and Teachers about TS

Educating classmates and teachers about Tourette Syndrome is essential to reduce stigma and promote understanding. Here are steps to take

1. **Presentation or Information Session** Organize a presentation or information session about TS for the student's classmates, teachers, and school staff. You can invite a guest speaker, such as a TS expert or a representative from a TS organization.

2. **Educational Materials** Distribute educational materials, brochures, or pamphlets about TS to teachers, classmates, and their families.

3. **Inclusive Classroom Discussion** Create opportunities for classroom discussions about TS and other neurodiverse conditions. Encourage questions and provide accurate, age-appropriate information.

4. **Storytelling** Share personal stories or experiences related to TS to humanize the condition and foster empathy.

5. **School Assemblies** If appropriate, consider organizing school assemblies or events dedicated to raising awareness about TS and other neurodiverse conditions.

6. **Online Resources** Share links to reputable online resources and videos that provide information and real-life stories about TS.

7. **Poster Campaign** Create posters or visual displays around the school to inform students about TS and promote acceptance.

8. **Peer Support Programs** Implement peer support programs that pair students with TS with "TS Ambassadors" who can help educate their peers about the condition.

By taking these steps, you can create a more inclusive and supportive school environment that fosters empathy, reduces stigma, and enhances understanding of Tourette Syndrome.

How can teachers support students with TS?

Teachers can support students with Tourette Syndrome (TS) in several ways to help them succeed in the classroom and manage their tics. Here are some strategies that teachers can use

Create a supportive environment Teachers can create a supportive and understanding environment by educating themselves and their students about TS. They can also encourage open communication and provide reassurance that tics are not a reflection of the student's intelligence or ability.

Accommodate tics Teachers can accommodate tics by allowing students to take breaks when needed, providing a quiet area for them to work, or giving them extra time to complete tasks. Teachers can also encourage students to use tic-management strategies such as deep breathing, relaxation techniques, or tic-reducing exercises.

Minimize stress Teachers can help minimize stress for students with TS by providing a structured and predictable routine, breaking down tasks into smaller steps, and offering positive reinforcement for their efforts.

Provide individualized support Teachers can provide individualized support by working with the student to develop a tic management plan that is tailored to their needs. This may include providing extra support during times when tics are severe, offering adaptations to the curriculum, or providing additional resources such as counseling or occupational therapy.

Encourage self-advocacy Teachers can encourage students with TS to self-advocate by teaching them how to explain their tics to their peers, advocating for their own needs, and seeking help when needed.

Educate peers Teachers can educate peers about TS and its effects on the student, which can help reduce stigma and promote understanding and acceptance.

Offer counseling Teachers can offer counseling or refer students to counseling services to help them cope with the emotional and social effects of TS.

Provide opportunities for movement Teachers can provide opportunities for students with TS to engage in physical activity, such as stretching, jumping jacks, or other movement-based activities, to help them manage their tics.

Encourage organization and planning Teachers can encourage students with TS to use organizational tools, such as planners or to-do lists, to help them stay on track and manage their time effectively.

Offer extra help Teachers can offer extra help to students with TS, such as tutoring or extra time to complete assignments, to help them succeed academically.

By using these strategies, teachers can help students with TS feel supported, confident, and successful in the classroom.

What resources are available for teachers to educate themselves about TS?

Educating yourself about Tourette Syndrome (TS) as a teacher is an important step in supporting students with TS effectively. Here are some valuable resources to help you learn more about TS:

1. **Tourette Association of America (TAA)** The TAA offers a wide range of educational resources and materials. Their website provides comprehensive information on TS, including webinars, fact sheets, and publications for educators.

2. **Centers for Disease Control and Prevention (CDC)** The CDC's "Learn More About Tourette Syndrome" page offers a concise overview of TS, its symptoms, and diagnosis. It also provides links to additional resources.

3. **National Institute of Neurological Disorders and Stroke (NINDS)** NINDS offers detailed information about TS, including research updates and treatment options.

4. **Books** There are several books available for educators that provide in-depth information about TS and practical strategies for supporting students. Consider titles like "Educators Guide to Teaching Students with Tourette Syndrome" by Woodbine House or "Tourette Syndrome A Practical Guide for Teachers, Parents and Carers" by London South Bank University.

5. **Online Courses** Some organizations, such as the TAA, offer online courses specifically designed for educators and school professionals. These courses cover the basics of TS, classroom strategies, and accommodations.

6. **Local TS Support Groups** Many regions have local TS support groups that hold meetings and events where you can connect with others and gain insights from experienced educators.

7. **Conferences and Workshops** Attend conferences, workshops, or training sessions on TS when available. These events often feature expert speakers and practical advice for educators.

8. **Professional Development** Contact your school district or educational institutions for information on professional development opportunities related to TS and other neurodiverse conditions.

9. **Online Forums and Communities** Join online forums and communities focused on education and special needs. These platforms can provide a space for discussion and sharing of knowledge and experiences.

10. **School Counselors and Special Education Teams** Collaborate with school counselors, special education teams, and colleagues who have experience working with students with TS. They can offer guidance and support.

By taking advantage of these resources, you can enhance your understanding of TS and develop effective strategies for creating an inclusive and supportive classroom environment for students with TS.

Chapter 7

Tourette Syndrome in the Workplace

How can employers support employees with TS?

Employers can support employees with Tourette Syndrome (TS) in several ways to create a more inclusive and supportive work environment. Here are some suggestions

Education and awareness Provide information and resources about TS to all employees to raise awareness and understanding of the condition. This can help reduce stigma and promote a more supportive work environment.

Accommodations Provide reasonable accommodations to help employees with TS perform their job duties effectively. This may include flexible work arrangements, modified work schedules, or assistive technology.

Supportive work environment Encourage a supportive work environment where employees with TS feel comfortable discussing their needs and concerns. This can include providing a private area for employees to take breaks or manage their tics, or offering flexible work arrangements to accommodate medical appointments.

Anti-discrimination policies Implement anti-discrimination policies that protect employees with TS from discrimination or harassment based on their condition.

Employee assistance programs Offer employee assistance programs (EAPs) that provide counseling, stress management, or other support services to help employees with TS manage their condition.

Open communication Encourage open communication between employees with TS and their managers and coworkers. This can help identify any challenges or issues that may arise and provide support to address them.

Job modifications Consider job modifications that can help employees with TS perform their job duties more effectively. This may include modifying job tasks, providing additional training, or adjusting work schedules.

Support for mental health Recognize that TS can have a significant impact on mental health and well-being. Provide support for employees with TS to access mental health resources, such as counseling or therapy, to help them manage stress and anxiety.

Flexible work arrangements Consider offering flexible work arrangements, such as telecommuting or flexible hours, to help employees with TS manage their condition.

Employee engagement Encourage employee engagement and participation in activities that promote well-being and inclusivity. This can help create a more supportive work environment for employees with TS.

By implementing these strategies, employers can create a more supportive work environment for employees with TS, which can help them feel valued, included, and productive.

Reasonable Accommodations for Employees with Tourette Syndrome (TS)

Reasonable accommodations are essential for ensuring that employees with Tourette Syndrome (TS) have equal opportunities in the workplace. The specific accommodations needed can vary depending on the individual's symptoms and challenges. Here are some common accommodations

1. **Flexible Work Schedule** Allow flexibility in work hours or breaks to accommodate the individual's needs, especially during periods of heightened tics or increased stress.

2. **Telecommuting** If possible, allow employees to work from home, which can reduce the stress and social interactions in the office that may exacerbate tics.

3. **Private Workspace** Provide a private workspace or allow the employee to use noise-cancelling headphones to reduce distractions and minimize the impact of tics on colleagues.

4. **Flexible Leave Policies** Offer flexible leave options, including sick leave or personal days, for days when tics are severe or when medical appointments are necessary.

5. **Job Restructuring** Adjust job tasks or responsibilities to accommodate the employee's strengths and reduce the impact of tics on performance.

6. **Assistive Technology** Provide or subsidize assistive technology or software that can help the employee manage tasks more effectively.

7. **Sensitivity Training** Conduct sensitivity training for colleagues and supervisors to increase awareness and understanding of TS, reducing potential stigma and misconceptions.

8. **Career Development Opportunities** Ensure that employees with TS have equal access to career development opportunities, including promotions and training.

9. **Access to Healthcare Benefits** Provide comprehensive healthcare benefits to cover the cost of therapy or medications related to TS.

10. **Written Communication** When possible, use written communication or emails for instructions or feedback to reduce face-to-face interactions.

11. **Appropriate Seating** Allow the employee to choose a comfortable and less noticeable seating arrangement to minimize social anxiety.

Promoting Education and Awareness about TS in the Workplace

Employers can take several steps to promote education and awareness about TS in the workplace

1. **Educational Workshops** Organize workshops or seminars on TS to help employees and supervisors understand the condition, its challenges, and the importance of support.

2. **Diversity and Inclusion Programs** Include TS and other neurodiverse conditions in diversity and inclusion programs to create a more inclusive workplace.

3. **Resource Materials** Provide informational materials about TS, including brochures or posters, in common areas.

4. **Communication Channels** Establish open channels for employees to discuss their needs and request accommodations in a safe and non-discriminatory manner.

5. **Accessibility Policies** Develop and communicate policies and procedures for requesting accommodations, ensuring confidentiality and privacy.

6. **Regular Updates** Regularly update employees on TS-related policies, resources, and available accommodations.

Common Challenges for Employees with TS in the Workplace

Employees with TS may face various challenges in the workplace, including

1. **Social Stigma** TS-related tics can lead to social stigma or misunderstandings among colleagues.

2. **Reduced Productivity** Tics can disrupt focus and productivity, leading to challenges in meeting job expectations.

3. **Increased Stress** Stress in the workplace can exacerbate tics, creating a cycle of increased anxiety and more tics.

4. **Social Anxiety** Employees with TS may experience social anxiety due to concerns about others' reactions to their tics.

5. **Accommodation Denial** Challenges may arise if employers fail to provide necessary accommodations or if employees do not disclose their condition.

6. **Reduced Job Satisfaction** The perception of a lack of understanding or support in the workplace can lead to reduced job satisfaction.

By implementing reasonable accommodations and promoting education and awareness, employers can create a more inclusive and supportive work environment for employees with TS, helping them overcome these challenges and thrive in their careers.

What resources are available for employers and employees with TS?

There are several resources available for employers and employees with Tourette Syndrome (TS). Here are some resources that can be helpful

For Employers

- Job Accommodation Network (JAN) JAN offers a wealth of information on accommodations for employees with disabilities, including TS. Employers can use JAN's resources to learn about accommodations that can be made for employees with TS[5].

- Neurodiversity Hub The Neurodiversity Hub provides resources for employers to develop greater awareness of neurodivergent talent in the community and develop strategies to support them in their journey of increased awareness[2].

- Employer Assistance and Resource Network on Disability Inclusion (EARN) EARN provides resources and assistance to employers to recruit, hire, retain, and advance people with disabilities. Employers can use EARN's resources to learn about accommodations for employees with TS[4].

For Employees

- Tourette Association of America The Tourette Association of America provides resources and support for individuals with TS and their families. They offer information on accommodations that can be made in the workplace[1].

- Job Accommodation Network (JAN) JAN provides resources for employees with disabilities, including TS. Employees can use JAN's resources to learn about accommodations that can be made in the workplace[5].

- Forage Forage provides information on reasonable accommodations at work, including changes to a hiring process, work environment, or job responsibilities that allow an employee with a disability to apply for or do their job. They offer examples of reasonable accommodations and how to request them in your job search or at your first job[6].

It's important to note that these resources are not exhaustive, and employers and employees should seek out additional resources as needed. Employers and employees should also work together to find accommodations that work best for the individual with TS.

Citations

[1] https//handbook.tts.gsa.gov/general-information-and-resources/business-and-ops-policies/top-secret

[2] https//www.neurodiversityhub.org/resources-for-employers

[3] https//www.itic.org/policy/coronavirus-response/resources-for-businesses-employers

[4] https//askearn.org

[5] https//www.business.com/legal/business-accommodations-guide-employees/

[6] https//www.theforage.com/blog/basics/reasonable-accommodations

Resources for Employees with TS to Find Job Opportunities

Finding job opportunities for employees with Tourette Syndrome (TS) may involve using specific resources that cater to diverse needs. Here are some resources to consider:

1. **Disability-Specific Job Boards** Websites like Disability Job Exchange, Recruit Disability, or the Job Accommodation Network (JAN) list job openings from employers specifically looking to hire individuals with disabilities.

2. **Job Placement Agencies** Reach out to job placement agencies that specialize in working with individuals with disabilities. They can assist in matching your skills and needs to suitable employers.

3. **Government Assistance Programs** Many countries have government programs and agencies that help individuals with disabilities find employment. In the United States, the Ticket to Work program can be a valuable resource.

4. **Local and National Disability Organizations** Organizations like the Tourette Association of America often provide job placement assistance and support for individuals with TS.

5. **Professional Networks** Join or explore professional networks and associations that focus on your field of expertise. These networks can help you access job opportunities and connect with potential employers who value diversity and inclusion.

6. **Online Job Search Engines** Utilize mainstream job search engines, but use filters to search for employers who promote diversity and inclusion.

7. **Career Development Centers** Many universities and colleges have career development centers that can provide guidance and resources for job seekers with disabilities.

Creating a More Inclusive Workplace for Employees with TS

Employers can take several steps to create a more inclusive workplace for employees with Tourette Syndrome

1. **Education and Training** Offer training and educational programs to all employees to increase awareness and understanding of TS and neurodiversity.

2. **Anti-Discrimination Policies** Implement clear anti-discrimination policies that prohibit any form of discrimination against employees with TS or other disabilities.

3. **Reasonable Accommodations** Develop processes for providing reasonable accommodations, and ensure that employees are aware of their rights in this regard.

4. **Mentoring and Support** Create mentoring programs or provide access to support networks for employees with TS, connecting them with colleagues who can offer guidance and understanding.

5. **Flexible Work Arrangements** Offer flexible work arrangements, including remote work or flexible hours, to accommodate the needs of employees with TS.

6. **Open Communication** Encourage open communication between employees and management, creating a culture where employees feel comfortable discussing their needs and challenges.

7. **Equal Opportunities** Ensure that employees with TS have equal opportunities for professional development, promotions, and career advancement.

Best Practices for Hiring Employees with TS

When hiring employees with Tourette Syndrome, consider the following best practices

1. **Inclusive Job Descriptions** Craft job descriptions and requirements that are inclusive and focused on skills and qualifications rather than perceived limitations.

2. **Interview Accommodations** Be prepared to provide accommodations during the interview process, such as allowing written responses or adjusting the interview format if needed.

3. **Anti-Bias Training** Train interviewers and hiring managers to recognize and address unconscious bias during the hiring process.

4. **Transparent Process** Be transparent about the hiring process and expectations, ensuring that candidates with TS understand the process and their rights.

5. **Collaboration** Collaborate with disability organizations and job placement agencies to identify candidates with TS who may be a good fit for your organization.

6. **Trial Periods** Consider offering trial periods or internships that allow candidates to showcase their skills and potential before committing to full-time employment.

7. **Feedback Mechanism** Establish a feedback mechanism for employees to express their needs, concerns, or suggestions related to the hiring and onboarding process.

By implementing these practices, employers can create an inclusive and supportive workplace where employees with TS can thrive and contribute to their full potential.

Chapter 8

Tourette Syndrome and Relationships

How does TS affect romantic relationships?

Tourette Syndrome (TS) can have a significant impact on romantic relationships, as it can affect the individual's ability to communicate, socialize, and engage in intimate relationships. Here are some ways in which TS can affect romantic relationships

Communication challenges People with TS may experience difficulty with verbal communication, which can lead to misunderstandings and conflicts in romantic relationships. They may have trouble expressing their thoughts and feelings, or they may experience difficulty understanding their partner's communication.

Social anxiety TS can cause individuals to experience social anxiety, which can make it challenging for them to engage in social situations, including romantic relationships. They may feel self-conscious about their tics or worried about being judged by their partner.

Emotional regulation TS can affect an individual's ability to regulate their emotions, which can lead to mood swings, irritability, and emotional outbursts. This can be challenging for romantic partners, who may struggle to understand and support their loved one.

Trust issues People with TS may have difficulty trusting their romantic partners due to their condition. They may worry that their partner will not accept them or that they will be judged for their tics.

Stigma and discrimination Unfortunately, there is still a lot of stigma and discrimination surrounding TS, which can affect romantic relationships. Partners may feel embarrassed or ashamed to be in a relationship with someone who has TS, or they may receive negative reactions from friends and family.

Limited dating pool Due to the challenges associated with TS, people with the condition may have a limited dating pool. They may find it difficult to find someone who is willing to accept and support them.

Self-esteem issues TS can affect an individual's self-esteem and confidence, which can make it challenging for them to form healthy romantic relationships. They may feel like they are not good enough or that they are a burden to their partner.

Difficulty with intimacy TS can affect an individual's ability to engage in intimate relationships, as they may experience difficulty with physical touch or may have tics that make it challenging to engage in sexual activity.

Misconceptions about TS There are many misconceptions about TS, which can affect romantic relationships. Partners may believe that TS is a sign of weakness or that it is something that can be controlled. Education and awareness are key to dispelling these misconceptions.

Support and understanding Despite the challenges associated with TS, many people with the condition are able to form successful romantic relationships. It is important for partners to understand and support their loved one, and to seek out resources and information to help them navigate the challenges associated with TS.

It's important to note that every person with TS is unique, and the impact of the condition on romantic relationships can vary widely. With understanding, support, and communication, many people with TS are able to form fulfilling and meaningful romantic relationships.

Improving communication skills in a romantic relationship, particularly when one partner has Tourette Syndrome (TS), is essential for maintaining a healthy and supportive connection. Here are some strategies to enhance communication and manage social anxiety in such relationships

Open and Honest Communication

- Establish a foundation of open and honest communication. Both partners should feel comfortable discussing their needs, concerns, and emotions.
- Encourage each other to express thoughts and feelings without judgment or criticism.
- Discuss TS-related challenges and the impact it may have on the relationship.

Education and Awareness

- Educate both partners about TS to enhance understanding. Knowledge can reduce misconceptions and promote empathy.
- Share reliable resources, articles, or books about TS to ensure that both partners have accurate information.

Active Listening

- Practice active listening by giving your partner your full attention when they're speaking.
- Repeat back what you've heard to ensure you've understood correctly, and validate your partner's feelings and experiences.

Empathy and Support

- Show empathy and support for your partner's experiences, including their challenges with TS.
- Demonstrate understanding and willingness to help when needed.

Patience and Tolerance

- Recognize that tics may become more prominent during stressful situations or emotional conversations. Be patient and understanding during these moments.
- Cultivate tolerance for the tics and other TS-related symptoms, understanding that they are involuntary.

Conflict Resolution

- Develop healthy conflict resolution skills. Address disagreements calmly and respectfully.
- Focus on the issues at hand, rather than personal attacks or criticisms.

Social Anxiety Management

- Encourage your partner to engage in stress-reduction techniques to manage social anxiety. These may include relaxation exercises, mindfulness, or therapy.
- Accompany your partner to social events to provide support and reduce anxiety.

Seek Professional Help

- Consider couples therapy or counseling to work through challenges, improve communication, and develop strategies for managing TS-related issues in the relationship.

Support Groups and Resources for Partners

- Look for support groups or organizations that focus on TS and relationships. The Tourette Association of America may provide resources and connections.
- Seek out online communities or forums where partners of individuals with TS can share experiences, advice, and support.

In a romantic relationship where one partner has TS, understanding, communication, and empathy are key. Both partners must work together to create an environment where the challenges of TS can be managed, and the relationship can thrive. Remember that every relationship is unique, and it may take time and effort to find the strategies and communication styles that work best for you both.

How does TS affect friendships and family relationships?

Tourette Syndrome (TS) can have a significant impact on friendships and family relationships. Here are some ways in which TS can affect these relationships

Social isolation People with TS may experience social isolation due to their condition. They may feel embarrassed or self-conscious about their tics, which can lead them to avoid social situations or withdraw from social interactions. This can lead to feelings of loneliness and isolation, which can affect their relationships with friends and family.

Stigma and discrimination Unfortunately, there is still a lot of stigma and discrimination surrounding TS. Friends and family members may not understand the condition, or they may have misconceptions about it. This can lead to feelings of embarrassment, shame, or anger, which can strain relationships.

Difficulty with communication TS can affect an individual's ability to communicate effectively. They may have difficulty expressing themselves, or they may experience difficulty with verbal or nonverbal communication. This can lead to misunderstandings and conflicts in relationships.

Emotional regulation TS can affect an individual's ability to regulate their emotions. They may experience mood swings, irritability, or emotional outbursts. This can be challenging for friends and family members, who may not know how to support their loved one.

Limited understanding Friends and family members may not fully understand the condition, which can lead to frustration and misunderstandings. They may not realize that the individual's tics are not under their control, or they may not understand the impact of the condition on their daily life.

Support and accommodations Friends and family members may not know how to support their loved one with TS. They may not understand the need for accommodations, such as providing a quiet space for their loved one to relax or avoiding triggers that can exacerbate their tics.

Impact on siblings If an individual with TS has siblings, the condition can affect them as well. Siblings may feel embarrassed or ashamed about their sibling's condition, or they may feel like they are unable to relate to their sibling.

Impact on parents TS can also affect the parents of an individual with the condition. They may feel guilty or responsible for their child's condition, or they may feel overwhelmed by the challenges of caring for a child with TS.

Difficulty with social events TS can make social events, such as parties or gatherings, challenging for individuals with the condition. They may feel

115

anxious or self-conscious about their tics, or they may have difficulty navigating social situations.

Impact on romantic relationships TS can also affect romantic relationships. Individuals with TS may have difficulty finding a partner who understands and accepts their condition, or they may experience discrimination or stigma from their partner's family and friends.

It's important to note that every individual with TS is unique, and the impact of the condition on friendships and family relationships can vary widely. However, with education, support, and understanding, individuals with TS can build strong and fulfilling relationships with their friends and family.

Supporting a friend or family member with Tourette Syndrome (TS) involves understanding their unique needs, offering empathy, and employing effective communication strategies. Here are some ways to better support someone with TS

Educate Yourself

- Learn about TS to gain a better understanding of the condition. Read books, articles, or attend workshops on TS to become informed.

Encourage Open Communication

- Create a safe space for your loved one to express their thoughts, feelings, and challenges related to TS.
- Ask questions and listen actively, demonstrating that you're interested in their experiences.

Show Empathy and Understanding

- Be empathetic and understanding when your loved one is dealing with tics or other TS-related symptoms. Show patience and compassion.

Be Supportive

- Offer support without judgment. Be there for your friend or family member, especially during difficult moments or when they're facing social challenges.

Respect Boundaries

- Respect your loved one's boundaries and personal space. Understand that there may be times when they need space or quiet.

Encourage Self-Advocacy

- Encourage your loved one to advocate for themselves and express their needs. This can include asking for specific accommodations when necessary.

Assist with Stress Management

- Support stress-reduction techniques, such as mindfulness, relaxation exercises, or seeking therapy if needed.

Participate in TS-Related Activities

- Attend TS-related events, workshops, or support groups together. This can help both you and your loved one connect with others facing similar challenges.

Encourage Independence

- Encourage your friend or family member to pursue their goals and interests. Independence and self-confidence are essential for individuals with TS.

Resources and Support Groups for Friends and Family

- The Tourette Association of America offers resources and support for friends and family members of individuals with TS. They may have local chapters or online communities you can join.

Strategies for Improving Communication

- Be patient and allow your loved one time to express themselves, especially when tics may momentarily disrupt their speech.
- Use non-verbal cues like nodding or maintaining eye contact to show that you're engaged and listening.
- Consider having regular check-ins to discuss how they're feeling and if they need any support.
- Educate other friends and family members about TS to ensure a supportive and understanding network.
- Collaborate on strategies for managing TS-related challenges together.

Remember that each person with TS is unique, and their needs and preferences may differ. By being a supportive and empathetic friend or family member, you can contribute to their well-being and create a more inclusive and understanding environment.

What resources are available for people with TS and their loved ones?

There are several resources available for people with Tourette Syndrome (TS) and their loved ones, including:

National Tourette Association (NTA) The NTA is a non-profit organization that provides information, support, and advocacy for people with TS and their families. They offer a variety of resources, including educational materials, support groups, and a national conference.

Tourette Syndrome Foundation of Canada (TSFC) The TSFC is a non-profit organization that provides information, support, and advocacy for people with TS and their families in Canada. They offer a variety of resources, including educational materials, support groups, and a national conference.

Tourette Association of America (TAA) The TAA is a non-profit organization that provides information, support, and advocacy for people with TS and their families in the United States. They offer a variety of resources, including educational materials, support groups, and a national conference.

International Tourette Syndrome Association (ITSA) The ITSA is a non-profit organization that provides information, support, and advocacy for people with TS and their families worldwide. They offer a variety of resources, including educational materials, support groups, and a global conference.

Tourette Syndrome Clinics and Centers There are several specialized clinics and centers that provide diagnosis, treatment, and management services for people with TS. These clinics and centers often have a team of healthcare professionals, including neurologists, psychologists, and social workers, who specialize in TS.

Online Support Groups There are several online support groups and forums for people with TS and their loved ones. These groups provide a safe and supportive environment where individuals can share their experiences, ask questions, and connect with others who understand the challenges of living with TS.

Educational Resources There are a variety of educational resources available for people with TS and their loved ones, including books, videos, and online courses. These resources can help individuals better understand TS, its symptoms, and its impact on daily life.

Advocacy Organizations There are several advocacy organizations that work to raise awareness and promote understanding of TS. These organizations often provide resources, support, and advocacy for people with TS and their families.

Mental Health Professionals Mental health professionals, such as psychologists, psychiatrists, and social workers, can provide diagnosis, treatment, and management services for people with TS. They can also provide support and guidance for loved ones.

Local Support Groups Local support groups can provide a safe and supportive environment where individuals with TS and their loved ones can connect with others who are going through similar experiences. These groups can also offer educational resources, support, and advocacy.

It's important to note that each person's experience with TS is unique, and the resources that are most helpful will vary depending on individual circumstances. It's often helpful to work with a healthcare professional to develop a personalized treatment plan that addresses the individual's specific needs and goals.

Educational resources

Tourette Association of America (TAA) The Tourette Association of America (TAA) is a leading national organization dedicated to serving the TS community. Here is some information about the TAA

- **Mission** The TAA's mission is to make life better for all people affected by Tourette and Tic Disorders. They provide support, education, and advocacy.

- **Educational Resources** The TAA offers a wide range of educational resources for individuals with TS, their families, educators, and healthcare professionals. These resources include fact sheets, webinars, publications, and information about the latest research and treatments.

- **Support and Community** The TAA provides support through local chapters and online communities. They host events, support groups, and conferences where individuals with TS and their families can connect and share their experiences.

- **Advocacy** The TAA advocates for individuals with TS at the federal, state, and local levels to promote policies and practices that support the TS community.

- **Find Local Support Groups** The TAA's website includes a tool that can help you find local support groups in your area. These groups offer a space for individuals with TS and their loved ones to connect and share their experiences.

To find local support groups for people with TS in your area and access educational resources, you can visit the Tourette Association of America's website at https//tourette.org. There, you'll find a wealth of information and tools to connect with the TS community and access the support and resources you need.

Chapter 9

Tourette Syndrome and Mental Health

What are the most common mental health problems in people with TS?

People with Tourette Syndrome (TS) are at a higher risk for developing mental health problems compared to the general population. The most common mental health problems in people with TS include

Anxiety disorders Anxiety disorders are the most common mental health problem in people with TS. They may experience excessive worry, fear, or anxiety that interferes with their daily life.

Depression Depression is a common mental health problem in people with TS. They may experience feelings of sadness, hopelessness, and a loss of interest in activities they once enjoyed.

Attention Deficit Hyperactivity Disorder (ADHD) ADHD is a common comorbidity in people with TS. They may experience difficulty paying attention, sitting still, and controlling their impulses.

Obsessive-Compulsive Disorder (OCD) OCD is a common comorbidity in people with TS. They may experience recurring thoughts, compulsions, and rituals that they feel compelled to perform.

Social anxiety disorder Social anxiety disorder is a common problem in people with TS. They may experience excessive fear or anxiety in social situations, such as public speaking or interacting with strangers.

Panic disorder Panic disorder is a common problem in people with TS. They may experience recurring panic attacks, which are sudden episodes of intense fear or anxiety that can occur at any time.

Post-traumatic stress disorder (PTSD) PTSD is a common problem in people with TS. They may experience symptoms such as flashbacks, nightmares, and avoidance of triggers that remind them of a traumatic event.

Sleep disorders Sleep disorders are common in people with TS. They may experience difficulty falling or staying asleep, or they may have excessive sleepiness during the day.

Eating disorders Eating disorders, such as anorexia nervosa or bulimia nervosa, are not uncommon in people with TS. They may experience difficulties with food restriction, binge eating, or purging.

Substance use disorders Substance use disorders, such as alcohol or drug addiction, are not uncommon in people with TS. They may use substances as a way to cope with their tics or other mental health symptoms.

It's important to note that these are not mutually exclusive, and many people with TS will experience multiple mental health problems simultaneously. It's important for individuals with TS to receive comprehensive care from a mental health professional to address their specific needs and symptoms.

Individuals with Tourette Syndrome (TS) may experience various mental health challenges, such as anxiety, depression, and obsessive-compulsive symptoms. Here are some common treatments and strategies to address these mental health issues

Cognitive-Behavioral Therapy (CBT)

- CBT is a well-established therapeutic approach that can help individuals with TS manage anxiety and depressive symptoms. It focuses on identifying and challenging negative thought patterns and behaviors.

Medication

- Medication may be prescribed to manage symptoms of anxiety, depression, or obsessive-compulsive disorder (OCD). Antidepressants, anti-anxiety medications, or other psychotropic drugs may be considered. It's essential to work with a healthcare provider to find the most suitable medication.

Exposure and Response Prevention (ERP)

- ERP is a specific form of CBT that is effective in treating OCD. It involves exposing individuals to their obsessions and preventing the associated compulsions, ultimately reducing OCD symptoms.

Stress-Reduction Techniques

- Learning stress-reduction techniques such as mindfulness, relaxation exercises, and deep breathing can help individuals with TS manage anxiety and stress.

Support Groups

- Support groups for individuals with TS and related mental health issues can provide a space to share experiences, gain insights, and offer emotional support.

Psychoeducation

- Psychoeducation programs can help individuals and their families understand the nature of TS and its associated mental health challenges, reducing stigma and increasing coping skills.

Social Support

- Building a strong support network of friends and family members can be immensely helpful in managing mental health issues.

Finding Mental Health Professionals

To find mental health professionals who specialize in the specific needs of individuals with TS

- Start by seeking recommendations from your primary care physician or neurologist. They may be able to refer you to mental health experts with experience in TS.
- Contact the Tourette Association of America (TAA) for recommendations and resources related to mental health professionals.
- Utilize online directories provided by professional organizations, such as the American Psychological Association or the Anxiety and Depression Association of America.

- Research local mental health providers and inquire about their experience with TS and related conditions.

Support Groups and Online Communities

There are several support groups and online communities for individuals with TS and their mental health challenges

- The TAA offers support groups for individuals with TS and their families. Check their website for information on local chapters and online support options.
- Online forums and communities like Reddit and social media groups may provide spaces for individuals to connect and share their experiences.
- Consider local or national mental health organizations that focus on anxiety, depression, and OCD, as they may have resources and support groups for people with these conditions.

It's important to remember that seeking professional help and connecting with others who share similar experiences can be a valuable step toward managing mental health challenges in the context of TS.

How are mental health problems treated in people with TS?

Mental health problems in people with Tourette Syndrome (TS) can be treated using a combination of psychotherapy and medication. The specific treatment approach will depend on the individual's specific symptoms and needs.

Psychotherapy

Cognitive-behavioral therapy (CBT) CBT is a type of therapy that helps individuals identify and change negative thought patterns and behaviors that contribute to their mental health problems. It can be effective in treating anxiety, depression, and obsessive-compulsive disorder (OCD) in people with TS.

Exposure and response prevention (ERP) ERP is a type of therapy that involves gradually exposing individuals to situations or stimuli that trigger their tics, while teaching them ways to manage their responses. It can be effective in reducing tic severity and improving mental health symptoms.

Habit reversal training Habit reversal training is a type of therapy that helps individuals identify and replace negative habits (such as tics) with more positive ones. It can be effective in reducing tic severity and improving mental health symptoms.

Medication

Antipsychotics Antipsychotic medications, such as haloperidol, can be effective in reducing tic severity and improving mental health symptoms in people with TS.

Antidepressants Antidepressant medications, such as selective serotonin reuptake inhibitors (SSRIs), can be effective in treating depression, anxiety, and OCD in people with TS.

Dopamine blockers Dopamine blockers, such as risperidone, can be effective in reducing tic severity and improving mental health symptoms in people with TS.

Botulinum toxin Botulinum toxin injections can be effective in reducing tic severity and improving mental health symptoms in people with TS.

Other treatments

Deep brain stimulation Deep brain stimulation is a surgical procedure that involves implanting a device that delivers electrical impulses to specific areas of the brain. It can be effective in reducing tic severity and improving mental health symptoms in people with TS.

Transcranial magnetic stimulation (TMS) TMS is a non-invasive procedure that involves using magnetic fields to stimulate specific areas of the brain. It can be effective in reducing tic severity and improving mental health symptoms in people with TS.

It's important to note that the most effective treatment approach will depend on the individual's specific needs and symptoms. A healthcare professional can work with the individual to develop a personalized treatment plan that takes into account their unique circumstances.

Potential Side Effects of Antipsychotic Medications for TS

Antipsychotic medications are sometimes prescribed to manage tics in individuals with Tourette Syndrome (TS). While they can be effective, they may also come with potential side effects, including

1. **Weight Gain** Some antipsychotic medications can lead to weight gain, which may increase the risk of obesity and related health issues.

2. **Sedation** Drowsiness or sedation is a common side effect of antipsychotic drugs, which can affect alertness and concentration.

3. **Extrapyramidal Symptoms (EPS)** EPS are movement-related side effects that can include tremors, muscle stiffness, restlessness (akathisia), and tardive dyskinesia (involuntary movements of the face and body).

4. **Metabolic Changes** Antipsychotics can lead to changes in blood sugar levels, cholesterol, and triglycerides, potentially increasing the risk of diabetes and cardiovascular problems.

5. **Hormonal Effects** Some antipsychotics may affect hormone levels, leading to menstrual irregularities and breast enlargement in men (gynecomastia).

6. **Neurological Effects** Rarely, antipsychotics can cause neuroleptic malignant syndrome (NMS), a potentially life-threatening condition with symptoms like high fever, muscle rigidity, and altered mental status.

7. **Tardive Dyskinesia** This is a long-term side effect characterized by involuntary movements, particularly of the face, lips, and tongue.

It's important to work closely with a healthcare provider when considering antipsychotic medications for TS. They can help weigh the potential benefits against the risk of side effects and determine the most suitable treatment plan.

Deep Brain Stimulation (DBS) for TS

Deep Brain Stimulation (DBS) is an invasive neurosurgical procedure that has shown promise in treating severe cases of TS, particularly when other treatments have not been effective. In DBS, electrodes are implanted in specific areas of the brain, and these electrodes deliver electrical stimulation to modulate neural activity. Some key points about DBS for TS include

- **Effectiveness** DBS has been shown to reduce tic severity and improve overall quality of life in some individuals with TS.

- **Candidate Selection** DBS is typically considered for individuals with severe and debilitating tics that significantly affect daily functioning and quality of life.

- **Surgery** The procedure involves brain surgery, and there are potential risks and complications, including infection and hardware-related issues.

- **Ongoing Monitoring** After DBS, ongoing monitoring and adjustment of stimulation settings are necessary to optimize outcomes and manage potential side effects.

- **Long-Term Results** The long-term effects of DBS for TS are still being studied, and it may not be suitable for all individuals.

Alternative Treatments for TS

Besides psychotherapy and medication, alternative treatments and lifestyle strategies that may help manage TS and its associated symptoms include

1. **Mind-Body Techniques** Mindfulness, relaxation exercises, and yoga can help reduce stress and anxiety, which may exacerbate tics.

2. **Diet and Nutrition** Some individuals have reported improvements in tics with dietary changes, such as avoiding certain trigger foods or additives.

3. **Exercise** Regular physical activity can help manage stress and improve overall well-being.

4. **Biofeedback** Biofeedback techniques can teach individuals to control physiological functions that may affect tics.

5. **Occupational Therapy** Occupational therapy can help individuals develop strategies to cope with daily challenges and improve functioning.

6. **Support Groups** Connecting with others who have TS can provide emotional support and practical insights for managing the condition.

It's essential to work with a healthcare provider or specialist to explore the most appropriate treatment options and develop an individualized plan for managing TS. Alternative treatments should be considered as complementary to evidence-based approaches.

What resources are available for people with TS and mental health problems?

There are several resources available for people with Tourette Syndrome (TS) and mental health problems. Here are some of them

National Tourette Association (NTA) The NTA provides information, resources, and support for individuals with TS and their families. They offer a variety of services, including a helpline, online support groups, and educational materials.

Tourette Syndrome Foundation of Canada (TSFC) The TSFC provides information, resources, and support for individuals with TS and their families in Canada. They offer a variety of services, including a helpline, online support groups, and educational materials.

Tourette Association of America (TAA) The TAA provides information, resources, and support for individuals with TS and their families in the United States. They offer a variety of services, including a helpline, online support groups, and educational materials.

Mental Health America Mental Health America is a national organization that provides information, resources, and support for individuals with mental health conditions, including TS. They offer a variety of services, including a helpline, online support groups, and educational materials.

National Alliance on Mental Illness (NAMI) NAMI is a national organization that provides information, resources, and support for individuals with mental health conditions, including TS. They offer a variety of services, including a helpline, online support groups, and educational materials.

Substance Abuse and Mental Health Services Administration (SAMHSA) SAMHSA is a government agency that provides information, resources, and support for individuals with mental health and substance use disorders, including TS. They offer a variety of services, including a helpline, online support groups, and educational materials.

Centers for Disease Control and Prevention (CDC) The CDC provides information, resources, and support for individuals with TS and other neurodevelopmental disorders. They offer a variety of services, including educational materials, research updates, and information on treatment options.

World Health Organization (WHO) The WHO provides information, resources, and support for individuals with TS and other mental health conditions. They offer a variety of services, including educational materials, research updates, and information on treatment options.

Online support groups There are several online support groups and forums for individuals with TS and mental health problems. These groups provide a safe and supportive environment where individuals can connect with others who share similar experiences and challenges.

Professional organizations There are several professional organizations that provide information, resources, and support for individuals with TS and mental health problems. These organizations include the American Psychiatric Association, the American Psychological Association, and the National Association of Social Workers.

It's important to note that these resources are not exhaustive and there may be other resources available depending on your location and specific needs. It's always a good idea to consult with a healthcare professional or mental health expert for personalized advice and guidance.

Online Support Groups for Individuals with TS and Mental Health Problems

1. **Tourette Association of America (TAA) Online Community** The TAA offers an online community where individuals with TS and their families can connect, share experiences, and seek support. You can find it on their website.

2. **Reddit - r/Tourettes** The r/Tourettes subreddit is a community where individuals with TS and their loved ones discuss a wide range of topics, including mental health challenges. It can be a valuable space for peer support and sharing insights.

3. **PsychCentral's Obsessive-Compulsive and Related Disorders Forum** This forum provides a space for individuals with OCD, which is often comorbid with TS, to discuss their experiences and challenges.

Local Organizations and Support Groups

1. **Tourette Association of America (TAA) Local Chapters** The TAA has local chapters across the United States. These chapters often host support groups and events, allowing individuals with TS and their families to connect on a local level.

2. **NAMI (National Alliance on Mental Illness)** While not specific to TS, NAMI offers local chapters and support groups for individuals and families affected by mental health conditions. They may have resources and information related to managing mental health challenges.

3. **Local Hospitals and Mental Health Clinics** Many healthcare facilities host support groups for individuals with various mental

health conditions. Contact local hospitals and clinics to inquire about available resources.

Common Treatment Options for Individuals with TS and Mental Health Problems

Treatment for individuals with TS and comorbid mental health problems often includes a combination of the following approaches:

1. **Cognitive-Behavioral Therapy (CBT)** CBT can help individuals manage anxiety, depression, and OCD symptoms by identifying and challenging negative thought patterns and behaviors.

2. **Medication** Medication may be prescribed to manage symptoms of anxiety, depression, or OCD. This can include antidepressants, anti-anxiety medications, or other psychotropic drugs.

3. **Exposure and Response Prevention (ERP)** ERP is a specific form of CBT that focuses on treating OCD by exposing individuals to their obsessions and preventing the associated compulsions.

4. **Support Groups** Support groups provide a space for individuals to share their experiences and seek emotional support from peers facing similar challenges.

5. **Stress-Reduction Techniques** Learning stress-reduction techniques such as mindfulness, relaxation exercises, and deep breathing can help individuals manage anxiety and stress.

6. **Psychoeducation** Educational programs can help individuals and their families understand the nature of TS and its associated mental health challenges, reducing stigma and increasing coping skills.

7. **Social Support** Building a strong support network of friends and family members can be immensely helpful in managing mental health issues.

It's important to work with healthcare providers, therapists, and specialists to develop an individualized treatment plan that addresses both TS and any comorbid mental health conditions. Treatment plans may vary based on the specific needs and preferences of each individual.

Chapter 10

Living Well with Tourette Syndrome

Tips for coping with tics

Tourette Syndrome (TS) is a neurodevelopmental disorder characterized by involuntary movements and vocalizations, known as tics. While there is no cure for TS, there are various strategies that can help individuals manage their tics and improve their quality of life. Here are some tips for coping with tics

Understand your tics It's essential to understand your tics and their triggers. Keeping a tic journal can help you identify the times of day, situations, or emotions that trigger your tics. This knowledge can help you prepare for and manage your tics better.

Develop a tic management plan Work with your healthcare provider to create a tic management plan that suits your needs. This plan may include medications, therapy, or lifestyle changes. Sticking to your plan can help you manage your tics and improve your quality of life.

Practice relaxation techniques Stress and anxiety can exacerbate tics. Practicing relaxation techniques such as deep breathing, progressive muscle relaxation, or meditation can help you calm your mind and body, reducing tic severity.

Engage in physical activity Regular exercise can help reduce tic severity and improve overall health. Activities like yoga, swimming, or walking can be beneficial, as they promote relaxation and reduce stress.

Avoid stimulants Caffeine, nicotine, and other stimulants can worsen tics. Limiting or avoiding these substances can help reduce tic severity and improve sleep quality.

Seek support Living with TS can be challenging, both for the individual and their family members. Joining a support group or seeking counseling can help you cope with the emotional impact of TS.

Educate yourself and others Learn as much as you can about TS and its effects on your life. Educate your family, friends, and colleagues about TS to raise awareness and dispel misconceptions.

Focus on abilities, not disabilities While TS can present challenges, it's essential to focus on your strengths and abilities. Engage in activities that bring you joy and help you build self-esteem.

Try alternative therapies Some people with TS have found relief from alternative therapies like acupuncture, massage, or music therapy. These therapies may help reduce tic severity or improve overall well-being.

Stay positive Maintaining a positive attitude can help you cope with the challenges of TS. Surround yourself with supportive people, practice gratitude, and celebrate small victories.

Remember, managing TS is a journey, and it's essential to be patient and persistent. By following these tips and working with your healthcare provider, you can find ways to cope with your tics and improve your quality of life.

Alternative Therapies for Tourette Syndrome

In addition to traditional treatments, some individuals with Tourette Syndrome (TS) explore alternative therapies to complement their management plan. While the effectiveness of these therapies can vary, here are a few alternatives that some individuals have found helpful

1. **Acupuncture** Acupuncture involves the insertion of fine needles into specific points on the body. Some people with TS have reported reduced tic severity and improved well-being with acupuncture.

2. **Hypnotherapy** Hypnotherapy can be used to help individuals with TS manage tics, anxiety, and stress. It aims to promote relaxation and reduce tic frequency.

3. **Yoga and Meditation** Mindfulness-based practices like yoga and meditation can help individuals manage stress and anxiety, which can exacerbate tics. These techniques focus on relaxation and self-awareness.

4. **Nutritional Approaches** Some individuals explore dietary changes, such as eliminating certain trigger foods or additives, to manage tics. However, the impact of diet on TS varies among individuals.

5. **Biofeedback** Biofeedback techniques teach individuals to control physiological functions, potentially helping with tic management.

6. **Cannabidiol (CBD)** CBD, a non-psychoactive compound in cannabis, has been explored by some as a potential treatment for TS. Research is ongoing to determine its effectiveness.

It's crucial to consult with a healthcare provider before trying alternative therapies, as they can help assess their safety and potential benefits in your specific case.

Finding Support Groups for Tourette Syndrome

To find a support group for individuals with Tourette Syndrome, consider the following steps

1. **Tourette Association of America (TAA)** The TAA has local chapters and online support options. Visit their website to explore the resources available and find a local chapter near you.

2. **Online Communities** Explore online platforms, such as social media, forums, and websites, where individuals with TS and their families share their experiences and offer support.

3. **Local Mental Health Organizations** Contact local mental health organizations or hospitals to inquire about support groups for TS. These may be connected to larger mental health or neurological support networks.

4. **Schools and Universities** Schools and universities sometimes host support groups for individuals with TS or neurodiverse conditions. Reach out to educational institutions in your area for information.

5. **Healthcare Providers** Your healthcare provider, such as a neurologist or therapist, may have information about local support groups or be able to make recommendations.

Common Triggers for Tics in Individuals with Tourette Syndrome

Tics in individuals with TS can be triggered or exacerbated by various factors, including

1. **Stress** Emotional or environmental stress is a common trigger for tics.

2. **Anxiety** High levels of anxiety can lead to increased tic frequency and intensity.

3. **Excitement** Positive emotions, such as excitement or anticipation, can trigger tics in some cases.

4. **Illness or Fatigue** Physical illness or fatigue can make tics more prominent.

5. **Sensory Sensitivities** Certain sensory stimuli, like noise or specific textures, can trigger tics in some individuals.

6. **Concentration and Suppression** Trying to suppress tics or concentrating intensely on not ticing can lead to a "rebound" effect, where tics become more pronounced later.

Understanding personal triggers and developing strategies to manage them is an important part of living with TS. It's essential for individuals with TS and their families to work with healthcare professionals to develop a holistic management plan that includes coping strategies for triggers and stressors.

Tips for managing stress

Managing stress can be particularly challenging for individuals with Tourette Syndrome (TS), as they may experience increased anxiety and tic severity in response to stressful situations. However, there are several strategies that can help people with TS manage stress and improve their overall well-being. Here are some tips

Practice relaxation techniques Relaxation techniques such as deep breathing, progressive muscle relaxation, and visualization can help reduce stress and anxiety. These techniques can be especially helpful for individuals with TS who may experience muscle tension or other physical symptoms related to stress.

Exercise regularly Exercise is a great way to reduce stress and improve overall health. People with TS may find that activities like yoga, swimming, or walking help them manage stress and anxiety.

Use positive self-talk Positive self-talk involves replacing negative thoughts with positive, empowering ones. This can help individuals with TS manage stress and anxiety by promoting a more positive outlook.

Engage in hobbies and activities Engaging in enjoyable activities can help distract from stress and provide a sense of relaxation and enjoyment. People with TS may find that activities like drawing, painting, or playing music help them manage stress.

Seek support Stress can be more manageable when you have a support system. People with TS may find it helpful to talk to a therapist, support group, or trusted friends and family members about their stress and anxiety.

Practice mindfulness Mindfulness involves being present in the moment and focusing on your thoughts, feelings, and sensations without judgment. This can help individuals with TS manage stress and anxiety by promoting a greater sense of self-awareness and calm.

Use stress management techniques There are a variety of stress management techniques that can be helpful for individuals with TS, such as time management, problem-solving, and communication skills.

Take breaks It's important to take breaks and give yourself time to rest and recharge. People with TS may find that taking short breaks throughout the day helps them manage stress and anxiety.

Get enough sleep Lack of sleep can exacerbate stress and anxiety. People with TS may find that getting enough sleep helps them manage stress and improve their overall well-being.

Consider therapy Cognitive-behavioral therapy (CBT) is a type of therapy that can be helpful for individuals with TS in managing stress and anxiety. CBT can help individuals identify and change negative thought patterns and behaviors that contribute to stress and anxiety.

It's important to remember that everyone is different, and what works for one person may not work for another. It may take some experimentation to find the strategies that work best for you. It's also important to work with a healthcare provider to develop a plan that's tailored to your individual needs.

Cognitive-Behavioral Therapy (CBT) for Managing Stress and Anxiety

Cognitive-Behavioral Therapy (CBT) is a widely used and evidence-based therapeutic approach that can be highly effective for individuals with Tourette Syndrome (TS) who experience stress and anxiety. Here's how CBT can help

1. **Identifying Thought Patterns** CBT involves identifying negative thought patterns or cognitive distortions that contribute to stress and anxiety. These distortions can include catastrophic thinking, overgeneralization, or all-or-nothing thoughts.

2. **Challenging Irrational Beliefs** Once identified, individuals work with a therapist to challenge and reframe irrational beliefs. They learn to question the accuracy and validity of their anxious thoughts.

3. **Behavioral Strategies** CBT also addresses behaviors that may reinforce anxiety. Individuals learn to recognize avoidance behaviors and gradually confront situations they fear, reducing anxiety over time.

4. **Relaxation Techniques** CBT often incorporates relaxation techniques to manage physical and emotional symptoms of stress and anxiety. These techniques can include deep breathing, progressive muscle relaxation, and guided imagery.

5. **Skill Building** CBT teaches individuals practical skills to manage stress and anxiety. These skills may include problem-solving, time management, and assertiveness training.

6. **Exposure and Response Prevention (ERP)** For individuals with TS who have co-occurring Obsessive-Compulsive Disorder (OCD), CBT may include ERP, a specific technique that helps individuals confront obsessive thoughts without engaging in compulsive behaviors.

Relaxation Techniques for Individuals with Tourette Syndrome

Relaxation techniques can be particularly helpful for managing the stress and anxiety associated with TS. Here are some relaxation methods that individuals with TS may find beneficial

1. **Deep Breathing** Slow, deep breaths can calm the nervous system. Practice inhaling slowly through your nose, holding for a few seconds, and exhaling through your mouth.

2. **Progressive Muscle Relaxation (PMR)** PMR involves tensing and then relaxing different muscle groups. This helps release physical tension and promote relaxation.

3. **Mindful Breathing** Mindfulness techniques encourage you to focus on your breath and the present moment. By paying attention to your breath without judgment, you can reduce anxiety.

4. **Guided Imagery** Visualization exercises can transport you to a calming and serene place in your mind. Visualize yourself in a tranquil setting, and focus on the details to induce relaxation.

5. **Yoga and Tai Chi** These mind-body practices combine physical movement with relaxation and mindfulness, helping reduce stress and anxiety.

Incorporating Mindfulness into Daily Routine

Mindfulness is a practice that involves paying deliberate attention to the present moment without judgment. It can be particularly useful for individuals with TS to manage stress and anxiety. Here's how to incorporate mindfulness into your daily routine

1. **Start with Short Sessions** Begin with short mindfulness sessions, even just a few minutes a day. Gradually increase the duration as you become more comfortable with the practice.

2. **Mindful Breathing** Take moments to focus on your breath. Inhale and exhale slowly, paying attention to the sensation of each breath.

3. **Mindful Eating** Pay close attention to the flavors, textures, and aromas of your meals. Eating mindfully can help reduce stress and enhance your connection to the present moment.

4. **Body Scan** Dedicate time to scan your body for areas of tension. Focus on relaxing and releasing tension in each body part.

5. **Mindful Walking** During walks, concentrate on each step, the feeling of your feet touching the ground, and the sounds of your surroundings.

6. **Mindful Moments** Integrate mindfulness into daily activities, such as washing dishes, taking a shower, or waiting in line. Use these moments to be fully present.

Remember that mindfulness is a skill that improves with practice. By incorporating it into your daily routine, you can enhance your ability to manage stress and anxiety, as well as reduce the impact of tics and other TS-related symptoms.

Tips for advocating for yourself

Educate yourself Learn as much as you can about TS, its symptoms, and its impact on your life. This will help you understand your needs and rights, and enable you to advocate for yourself more effectively.

Be assertive Speak up for yourself and express your needs clearly and respectfully. Practice using assertive language, such as "I need" or "I want," and be specific about what you are asking for.

Build a support network Surround yourself with people who understand and support you, such as family, friends, and healthcare providers. This network can provide emotional support, help you navigate challenges, and advocate for you when needed.

Be prepared to educate others Many people may not understand TS or its impact on your life. Be prepared to educate them about your experiences and needs, and provide resources or information to help them understand better.

Advocate for accommodations If you need accommodations at school, work, or in other areas of life, advocate for them assertively and persistently. Explain your needs and why they are important for your success and well-being.

Seek out resources There are many resources available for people with TS, such as support groups, advocacy organizations, and online forums. Seek out these resources and use them to connect with others, find information, and advocate for yourself.

Be patient and persistent Advocating for yourself can be challenging, and it may take time to achieve your goals. Be patient and persistent, and don't give up if you encounter obstacles or setbacks.

Practice self-advocacy in daily life Practice self-advocacy in your daily life by speaking up for yourself, expressing your needs, and assertively asking for what you want. This will help you build confidence and skills that will benefit you in the long run.

Seek professional help If you are struggling with self-advocacy or need additional support, consider seeking help from a mental health professional or advocacy organization. They can provide you with guidance, resources, and support to help you advocate for yourself effectively.

Celebrate your successes Celebrate your successes, no matter how small they may seem. This will help you build confidence and motivation to continue advocating for yourself.

Remember, advocating for yourself is an ongoing process, and it's important to be patient, persistent, and assertive. By following these tips, you can effectively advocate for yourself and improve your quality of life.

Finding Support Groups and Advocacy Organizations for TS

1. **Tourette Association of America (TAA)** The TAA is the primary national organization dedicated to TS. They provide resources, support groups, and advocacy opportunities. Visit their website or contact them to find local chapters and events.

2. **Local Mental Health Organizations** Many local mental health organizations or community centers may host support groups for individuals with TS. Contact them to inquire about available resources.

3. **Online Communities** Explore online platforms, such as social media groups, forums, and websites, where individuals with TS and their families share experiences, offer support, and discuss advocacy efforts.

4. **Educational Institutions** Schools and universities may have support groups and resources for students with TS. Inquire about these resources at educational institutions in your area.

5. **Healthcare Providers** Healthcare providers, such as neurologists and therapists, may have information about local support groups or be able to make recommendations.

Common Challenges in Self-Advocacy for People with TS

Self-advocacy can be empowering, but it may also come with challenges for individuals with TS

1. **Stigma** Overcoming social stigma associated with TS can be difficult. Some people may lack awareness or understanding, leading to misconceptions and biases.

2. **Public Misconceptions** Dealing with misconceptions and societal misunderstandings can be frustrating, as TS is often misrepresented in media and popular culture.

3. **Tic-Related Obstacles** Tics may complicate self-advocacy, as they can be misunderstood or misinterpreted, making communication more challenging.

4. **Access to Services** Some individuals may face barriers in accessing appropriate healthcare, educational, or workplace accommodations.

5. **Emotional Impact** Advocating for oneself can be emotionally taxing, especially when facing resistance or discrimination.

Tips for Dealing with Setbacks or Obstacles in Self-Advocacy

1. **Educate Yourself** Equip yourself with knowledge about TS and its challenges. The more informed you are, the better you can advocate effectively.

2. **Build a Support Network** Seek support from family, friends, and fellow advocates who understand your journey and can offer guidance and encouragement.

3. **Use Your Voice** Don't hesitate to speak up and share your experiences with TS. Your personal stories can be powerful tools for raising awareness.

4. **Set Realistic Goals** Break down your advocacy efforts into achievable, manageable goals. Celebrate small victories along the way.

5. **Be Persistent** Self-advocacy often requires patience and persistence. Be prepared for resistance and setbacks, but don't let them deter you from your mission.

6. **Collaborate** Work with advocacy organizations, support groups, and allies who share your goals and can amplify your efforts.

7. **Seek Legal Advice** If you face discrimination or unfair treatment, consult legal experts who specialize in disability rights to understand your rights and options.

8. **Self-Care** Prioritize self-care to manage stress and maintain your physical and mental well-being. Advocacy can be demanding, so taking care of yourself is crucial.

9. **Raise Awareness** Participate in activities to raise awareness about TS, such as organizing events, writing articles, or giving presentations.

10. **Know When to Seek Help** If self-advocacy becomes overwhelming, seek help from professionals or advocates experienced in supporting individuals with TS.

Advocacy for oneself and for the TS community is a valuable and meaningful endeavor. By navigating challenges with resilience and determination, you can make a significant impact in promoting understanding and acceptance of TS while improving your own quality of life.

Resources for people with TS and their loved ones

There are several resources available for people with Tourette Syndrome (TS) and their loved ones. Here are some of the most helpful resources

Tourette Association of America (TAA) The TAA is a national organization that provides information, resources, and support for people with TS and their families. They offer a variety of services, including a helpline, online support groups, and educational materials.

Tourette Syndrome Foundation of Canada (TSFC) The TSFC is a Canadian organization that provides information, resources, and support for people with TS and their families. They offer a variety of services, including a helpline, online support groups, and educational materials.

International Tourette Syndrome Association (ITSA) ITSA is an international organization that provides information, resources, and support for people with TS and their families. They offer a variety of services, including a helpline, online support groups, and educational materials.

National Tourette Syndrome Awareness Month May is National Tourette Syndrome Awareness Month, which is a great time to raise awareness and educate others about TS. Many organizations and individuals use this month to share information, personal stories, and resources on social media and in their communities.

Tourette Syndrome Support Groups Joining a support group can be a great way to connect with others who understand what it's like to live with TS. Many support groups are available in person or online, and they offer a safe space to share experiences, ask questions, and get support.

Online Forums and Communities There are several online forums and communities dedicated to TS, where people can ask questions, share experiences, and connect with others who are going through similar challenges. Some popular online communities include the TS subreddit, Tourette Syndrome Forum, and TS Support Group.

Books and Documentaries There are several books and documentaries available that provide insight into the experiences of people with TS. Some popular books include "The Tourette Syndrome Handbook" by Dr. James F. Leckman and "Tourette Syndrome A Guide for the Newly Diagnosed" by Dr. Tammy L. Hesser. Some popular documentaries include "Tourette Syndrome A Life of Twitches and Squeaks" and "Tourette A Family's Quest for Normalcy."

Mental Health Professionals Finding a mental health professional who is knowledgeable about TS can be a great resource for people with the condition. Many therapists and counselors specialize in working with people with TS and can provide valuable guidance and support.

TS-Friendly Schools and Workplaces Creating TS-friendly schools and workplaces can make a big difference for people with TS. Many organizations offer resources and support for educators and employers who want to create a more inclusive environment for people with TS.

Research Studies Participating in research studies can be a great way to contribute to the understanding of TS and potentially improve treatments and outcomes. Many research studies are available, and they often offer compensation for participants.

These are just a few of the many resources available for people with TS and their loved ones. It's important to remember that each person's experience with TS is unique, and what works for one person may not work for another. It's often helpful to try out a few different resources to find the ones that work best for you.

Online Support Groups for TS

1. **Tourette Association of America (TAA) Online Community** The TAA hosts an online community where individuals with TS and their families can connect, share experiences, and seek support. You can access this community through the TAA's website.

2. **Reddit - r/Tourettes** The r/Tourettes subreddit is an online community where individuals with TS and their loved ones discuss a wide range of topics, share experiences, and offer support.

3. **Facebook Groups** There are several TS-related groups on Facebook where individuals with TS and their families gather to share their stories and support one another.

4. **DailyStrength - Tourette Syndrome Support Group** DailyStrength offers an online support group for individuals with TS. It's a platform for sharing experiences and finding emotional support.

Books and Documentaries about TS

1. **Book - "Front of the Class How Tourette Syndrome Made Me the Teacher I Never Had" by Brad Cohen** This memoir tells

the inspiring story of a man with TS who becomes an educator and advocate.

2. **Book - "Life's A Twitch! An Insider's Tale of Tourette Syndrome" by Tim Howard** In this book, the author, who has TS, shares his personal journey and experiences.

3. **Documentary - "I Have Tourettes But Tourettes Doesn't Have Me"** This documentary provides a personal and in-depth look at the lives of individuals living with TS.

4. **Documentary - "Twitch and Shout"** This documentary explores the lives of four individuals with TS, offering insights into their daily challenges and triumphs.

Finding Mental Health Professionals Specializing in TS

1. **Tourette Association of America (TAA)** The TAA can provide recommendations for healthcare providers, therapists, and specialists with experience in TS. Contact them for assistance.

2. **Ask for Referrals** Consult with your primary care physician, neurologist, or other healthcare providers. They may be able to refer you to mental health professionals who specialize in TS.

3. **Online Directories** Professional organizations, such as the American Psychological Association and the Anxiety and Depression Association of America, offer online directories to find qualified mental health professionals in your area.

4. **Local Mental Health Clinics and Hospitals** Reach out to local mental health clinics and hospitals to inquire about professionals who have experience in working with individuals with TS.

5. **University Medical Centers** Academic medical centers often have specialists who are knowledgeable about neurological and neuropsychiatric conditions, including TS.

6. **Telehealth Services** Given the availability of telehealth services, you can also consider online therapy platforms where you can access mental health professionals from the comfort of your home.

When seeking a mental health professional, it's essential to discuss your specific needs and ensure they have experience in working with TS or related conditions. A qualified and understanding mental health professional can provide effective support and treatment tailored to your individual situation.

Chapter 11

Tourette Syndrome in the Media

How has TS been portrayed in the media?

Tourette Syndrome (TS) has been portrayed in various ways in the media, ranging from accurate and respectful depictions to stereotypical and stigmatizing portrayals. Here are some examples

Accurate and respectful portrayals
    The film "The Imitation Game" (2014) tells the story of Alan Turing, a mathematician and computer scientist who had TS. The film portrays TS in a nuanced and respectful way, highlighting Turing's struggles with the condition and his determination to overcome it.
    The TV show "The Good Doctor" (2017-present) features a character with TS, Dr. Shaun Murphy, who is a brilliant surgeon. The show portrays TS in a positive light, highlighting the character's strengths and abilities despite his challenges.
    The documentary "Tourette Syndrome A Life of Twitches and Squeaks" (2012) follows the lives of several people with TS, showcasing their experiences and challenges in a respectful and informative way.

Stereotypical and stigmatizing portrayals
    The film "The Madwoman of Chaillot" (1969) features a character with TS who is portrayed as a stereotypical "mad scientist" with a wild, uncontrollable laugh.
    The TV show "The Simpsons" (1989-present) has a character named Ned Flanders who has TS. However, the show often portrays Flanders as a caricature, with his TS being used as a punchline for jokes.
    The film "Me, Myself & Irene" (2000) features a character with TS who is portrayed as a violent, aggressive person. The film perpetuates negative stereotypes about TS and reinforces harmful stigmas.

Overall, the media has a mixed record when it comes to portraying TS. While there have been some accurate and respectful portrayals, there have also been many stereotypical and stigmatizing depictions that perpetuate negative attitudes towards people with TS. It's important for the media to portray TS in a respectful and nuanced way, highlighting the experiences and challenges faced by people with the condition, and promoting greater understanding and acceptance.

Films and TV Shows Portraying TS

While accurate portrayals of Tourette Syndrome (TS) are relatively rare in mainstream media, there are a few notable examples

1. **"Front of the Class" (2008)** This TV movie is based on the life of Brad Cohen, who has TS and becomes a teacher. It provides an inspiring and authentic portrayal of his experiences.

2. **"The Tic Code" (1999)** This film explores the life of a jazz musician with TS. While it's a fictional story, it delves into the challenges and creativity of the character's experience.

3. **"Different Minds A Remarkable Story of Autism, Asperger's, and Tourette" (2011)** This documentary offers insights into the lives of individuals with various neurodiverse conditions, including TS.

Promoting Accurate and Respectful Portrayals of TS in the Media

1. **Raise Awareness** The first step in promoting accurate portrayals is to raise awareness about TS. Share information and personal stories to educate both the public and media professionals.

2. **Advocate for Inclusive Casting** Encourage the casting of actors with TS in roles that depict the condition. Authentic representation can lead to more accurate portrayals.

3. **Consult Experts** Filmmakers and writers should consult experts, individuals with TS, and advocacy organizations to ensure accurate depictions.

4. **Avoid Stereotypes** Promote narratives that go beyond stereotypes and showcase the diverse experiences of individuals with TS.

5. **Engage with Media Outlets** Contact media outlets, including TV networks and production companies, to express your interest in accurate and respectful portrayals of TS. Advocate for sensitivity in their content.

Organizations and Initiatives

1. **Tourette Association of America (TAA)** The TAA plays a vital role in advocating for accurate and respectful portrayals of TS in the media. They collaborate with content creators and provide resources on TS awareness.

2. **Media Advocacy Program** The TAA's Media Advocacy Program works to educate the media and promote responsible reporting and storytelling about TS.

3. **Film Festivals** Some film festivals, such as the ReelAbilities Film Festival, showcase films that focus on disability and neurodiversity, including TS.

4. **Social Media Campaigns** Join or support social media campaigns that aim to highlight the need for accurate and respectful portrayals of TS in the media.

5. **Content Ratings and Reviews** Encourage rating and review platforms to include assessments of media portrayals, promoting positive representations and flagging harmful stereotypes.

By actively participating in advocacy efforts, sharing your experiences, and supporting organizations that work toward better representation, you can contribute to the shift toward more accurate and respectful depictions of TS in the media.

What are the positive and negative effects of media portrayals of TS?

Media portrayals of Tourette Syndrome (TS) can have both positive and negative effects on the public's perception and understanding of the condition. Here are some of the potential effects

Positive effects

Increased awareness Media portrayals of TS can help raise awareness about the condition and educate the public about its symptoms, causes, and impact on individuals and families.

Reduced stigma Accurate and respectful media portrayals can help reduce stigma and stereotypes associated with TS, promoting greater understanding and acceptance of people with the condition.

Improved diagnosis and treatment Media portrayals can encourage people to seek medical attention if they suspect they or their family members may have TS, leading to earlier diagnosis and treatment.

Increased funding for research Media attention can raise awareness among policymakers and funding agencies, potentially leading to increased funding for research and treatment development.

Negative effects

Perpetuation of stereotypes Inaccurate or stereotypical media portrayals can reinforce negative attitudes and stereotypes about TS, perpetuating harmful stigmas and discrimination.

Misinformation Media portrayals that are inaccurate or sensationalized can spread misinformation about TS, leading to confusion and misconceptions among the public.

Exploitation Sensationalized media portrayals can exploit people with TS for entertainment value, reinforcing harmful stereotypes and potentially causing harm to individuals and families affected by the condition.

Increased anxiety and stress Media portrayals that emphasize the negative aspects of TS can create anxiety and stress for people with the condition, their families, and caregivers.

Overall, the impact of media portrayals of TS depends on the accuracy, respect, and sensitivity with which they are portrayed. Positive portrayals can promote greater understanding, reduce stigma, and improve diagnosis and treatment. Negative portrayals can perpetuate harmful stereotypes, spread misinformation, and cause harm to individuals and families affected by the condition.

Advocating for More Accurate Media Portrayals

Individuals and families affected by Tourette Syndrome (TS) can play a crucial role in advocating for more accurate media portrayals. Here's how you can get involved

1. **Raise Awareness** Start by raising awareness about TS and the importance of accurate media portrayals. Share information and personal stories through social media, blogs, and community events.

2. **Connect with Advocacy Organizations** Join or support organizations like the Tourette Association of America (TAA), which actively advocate for better media representation. These organizations often have advocacy campaigns and resources to help you get involved.

3. **Engage with Media Outlets** Reach out to media outlets, TV networks, and production companies to express your interest in accurate and sensitive portrayals of TS. Advocate for their responsibility in shaping public perceptions.

4. **Share Personal Stories** If you or your family is affected by TS, consider sharing your personal experiences with local and national media. Authentic narratives can have a profound impact on raising awareness.

5. **Consult with Experts** Encourage filmmakers, writers, and producers to consult with experts in TS and neuropsychiatric conditions to ensure accurate depictions.

Ensuring Sensitive and Informative Media Portrayals

To ensure that media portrayals of TS are sensitive and informative, follow these steps

1. **Educate Creators** Provide educational resources and offer to connect media professionals with experts in TS who can provide insights into the condition.

2. **Collaborate with Advocacy Organizations** Partner with organizations like the TAA to access guidance and support in creating accurate portrayals.

3. **Diverse Perspectives** Encourage media creators to feature a diverse range of characters with TS to reflect the varied experiences within the TS community.

4. **Avoid Stereotypes** Advocate for narratives that go beyond stereotypes and depict the multi-faceted experiences of individuals with TS.

5. **Screen Content** Consider hosting pre-release screenings or focus groups to gather feedback from individuals with TS and their families to ensure that the portrayal is sensitive and accurate.

6. **Listen to Feedback** Be open to feedback from the TS community and be willing to make necessary adjustments to content based on their input.

7. **Promote Inclusive Hiring** Encourage the inclusion of individuals with TS in key roles in the entertainment industry, both in front of and behind the camera.

By actively participating in advocacy efforts, sharing personal stories, and supporting organizations that work toward better representation, individuals and families can contribute to more accurate, sensitive, and informative media portrayals of TS.

How can we promote accurate and positive representations of TS in the media?

Promoting accurate and positive representations of Tourette Syndrome (TS) in the media is important for raising awareness and reducing stigma associated with the condition. Here are some ways to promote positive and accurate representations of TS in the media

Educate journalists and media professionals Provide information and resources to journalists and media professionals about TS, its symptoms, and its impact on individuals and families. This can help them to report on TS in a respectful and accurate manner.

Encourage positive storytelling Share positive stories and experiences of people with TS, highlighting their strengths, accomplishments, and contributions to society. This can help to counterbalance negative stereotypes and stigmatizing portrayals.

Provide media guidelines Develop and disseminate media guidelines for reporting on TS, emphasizing the importance of accuracy, respect, and sensitivity. This can help journalists and media professionals to avoid perpetuating negative stereotypes and stigmatizing language.

Engage with media organizations Reach out to media organizations and offer to provide expert advice and information on TS. This can help to ensure that media reports are accurate and respectful.

Use social media Utilize social media platforms to share positive and accurate information about TS, and to engage with journalists and media professionals. This can help to promote a more nuanced understanding of TS and counterbalance negative stereotypes.

Support media advocacy campaigns Participate in media advocacy campaigns that aim to promote positive and accurate representations of TS. This can help to raise awareness and reduce stigma associated with the condition.

Encourage diverse representation Encourage media representations of TS that reflect the diversity of the TS community, including different ages, genders, ethnicities, and backgrounds. This can help to promote a more inclusive and nuanced understanding of TS.

Provide media training Offer media training to people with TS and their families, helping them to share their stories and experiences in a way that is respectful and accurate.

Engage with influencers Partner with social media influencers who have TS or who are passionate about raising awareness about the condition. This can help to promote positive and accurate representations of TS to a wider audience.

Celebrate positive media representations Celebrate and promote positive media representations of TS, such as films, TV shows, or articles that portray TS in an accurate and respectful manner. This can help to reinforce positive stereotypes and promote greater understanding and acceptance of TS.

By taking these steps, we can promote positive and accurate representations of TS in the media, helping to reduce stigma and improve understanding of the condition.

Engaging with Media Organizations to Provide Expert Advice on TS

1. **Contact Media Outlets** Reach out to local and national media organizations through email, phone calls, or social media. Express your willingness to provide expert advice on TS for their programs or content.

2. **Offer Expertise** In your communications, highlight your expertise or the expertise of individuals within the TS community who are willing to provide insights into the condition. Explain how their perspectives can contribute to more accurate portrayals.

3. **Create a Network** Connect with organizations like the Tourette Association of America (TAA), which may already have established relationships with media outlets. Collaborating with these organizations can help you access more opportunities to provide expert advice.

Examples of Media Advocacy Campaigns Promoting Positive Representations of TS

1. **TAA's Media Advocacy Program** The TAA actively engages with media outlets to promote responsible reporting and storytelling about TS. They provide resources, toolkits, and opportunities for advocates to participate in media campaigns.

2. **Social Media Campaigns** Many individuals and organizations use social media platforms to launch campaigns that advocate for positive representations of TS in the media. By sharing stories, facts, and experiences, these campaigns aim to influence media content.

3. **"Touretteshero"** This is a UK-based initiative led by Jessica Thom, who has TS. The project challenges stereotypes and misconceptions about TS through creative and artistic means, including theater and social media.

Encouraging Diverse Representation of TS in the Media

1. **Advocate for Inclusive Casting** Encourage casting directors and producers to consider individuals with TS for roles that depict the condition. This authentic representation can help showcase the diversity of TS experiences.

2. **Collaborate with Diverse Voices** Work with writers, directors, and producers from diverse backgrounds who can bring their unique perspectives to stories involving TS.

3. **Story Development** Collaborate with writers and content creators to ensure that characters with TS have multi-dimensional and culturally diverse backgrounds, reflecting the experiences of the broader TS community.

4. **Consult with Diverse Experts** Ensure that individuals providing expert advice on TS come from diverse backgrounds to offer a range of experiences and insights.

5. **Diversity in Production Crews** Advocate for diverse representation in production crews, including camera operators, directors, and costume designers, to contribute to a more holistic portrayal of TS.

6. **Address Intersectionality** Recognize that individuals with TS may also belong to various demographic groups. Encourage storytelling that explores the intersectionality of TS with other aspects of identity, such as race, gender, or sexual orientation.

By engaging with media organizations, participating in advocacy campaigns, and advocating for diverse representation, you can help promote more authentic, inclusive, and positive media portrayals of Tourette Syndrome.

Chapter 12

The Future of Tourette Syndrome Research and Treatment

What are the most promising areas of research on TS?

There are several promising areas of research on Tourette Syndrome (TS), including

Genetics Researchers are studying the genetic factors that contribute to the development of TS, with the goal of identifying new targets for treatment.

Brain imaging Advanced brain imaging techniques, such as functional magnetic resonance imaging (fMRI), are being used to study the brain mechanisms underlying TS. This research may lead to new treatments that target specific brain regions or networks.

Neurostimulation Techniques such as deep brain stimulation (DBS) and transcranial magnetic stimulation (TMS) have shown promise in treating TS. Researchers are working to improve the effectiveness and safety of these treatments.

Gene therapy Scientists are exploring the use of gene therapy to treat TS. This approach involves inserting a healthy copy of a gene into a person's cells to replace a faulty gene that may be contributing to the condition.

Environmental factors Researchers are studying the role of environmental factors, such as stress and anxiety, in triggering TS symptoms. Understanding these factors may help develop new treatments that focus on managing stress and anxiety.

Immunotherapy Some research suggests that TS may be linked to abnormalities in the immune system. Immunotherapy, which uses the body's immune system to fight disease, may be a promising area of research for TS treatments.

Non-invasive brain stimulation Techniques such as transcranial direct current stimulation (tDCS) and transcranial alternating current stimulation (tACS) have shown promise in treating TS symptoms. These non-invasive techniques may offer a safer and more accessible alternative to DBS.

Personalized medicine Researchers are working to develop personalized treatments for TS that take into account an individual's unique genetic and environmental factors. This approach may lead to more effective and targeted treatments.

Virtual reality therapy Virtual reality (VR) therapy is being explored as a
potential treatment for TS. VR may help individuals with TS confront and
overcome triggers for their tics in a controlled environment.

Mindfulness-based interventions Mindfulness-based interventions, such as
meditation and yoga, have shown promise in reducing stress and anxiety in
individuals with TS. These interventions may also help reduce tic severity.

It's important to note that these are just a few examples of promising areas of
research, and that the field of TS research is constantly evolving. New
breakthroughs and discoveries may lead to additional promising areas of
research in the future.

Latest advancements in gene therapy for TS

Gene therapy is a promising new approach to treating TS, but it is still in the
early stages of development. The goal of gene therapy is to deliver a healthy
copy of the TS-causing gene to the brain. This could potentially cure TS or
significantly reduce its symptoms.

One of the most promising gene therapy approaches for TS is called AAV-
AS10 This therapy uses a harmless virus to deliver a healthy copy of the TS-
causing gene to the brain. AAV-AS101 has been shown to be safe and effective
in animal studies, and it is currently in Phase 1 clinical trials in humans.

Another promising gene therapy approach for TS is called CRISPR-Cas9 gene
editing. CRISPR-Cas9 is a powerful tool that can be used to make precise
changes to DNA. Scientists are using CRISPR-Cas9 to develop gene therapies
that can correct the genetic mutation that causes TS. CRISPR-Cas9 gene
editing is still in the early stages of development, but it has the potential to be
a very effective treatment for TS.

How virtual reality therapy can help individuals with TS manage their symptoms

Virtual reality (VR) therapy is a new and innovative approach to treating a variety of mental health conditions, including TS. VR therapy works by immersing the user in a simulated environment that can be used to teach new skills, challenge negative thoughts and behaviors, and provide exposure to feared situations.

VR therapy has been shown to be effective in reducing the symptoms of TS, such as tics and obsessive-compulsive symptoms. One study found that VR therapy was more effective in reducing tics than traditional cognitive-behavioral therapy (CBT). Another study found that VR therapy was effective in reducing obsessive-compulsive symptoms in people with TS.

VR therapy is a safe and well-tolerated treatment for TS. It is also a relatively new treatment, so more research is needed to confirm its long-term efficacy. However, the results of existing studies suggest that VR therapy is a promising new treatment for TS.

Ongoing clinical trials for TS treatments in the field of neurostimulation

There are several ongoing clinical trials for TS treatments in the field of neurostimulation. Neurostimulation is a type of therapy that uses electrical or magnetic currents to stimulate the brain.

One type of neurostimulation that is being investigated for TS is called deep brain stimulation (DBS). DBS involves implanting electrodes into the brain and delivering electrical currents to specific areas of the brain. DBS has been shown to be effective in reducing the symptoms of some other neurological disorders, such as Parkinson's disease and essential tremor.

Another type of neurostimulation that is being investigated for TS is called transcranial magnetic stimulation (TMS). TMS is a non-invasive type of neurostimulation that uses magnetic fields to stimulate the brain. TMS has been shown to be effective in reducing the symptoms of some other mental health conditions, such as depression and OCD.

Clinical trials are currently underway to investigate the safety and efficacy of DBS and TMS for the treatment of TS. The results of these trials will help to determine whether neurostimulation is a viable treatment option for TS.

Here are some examples of ongoing clinical trials for TS treatments in the field of neurostimulation

- A Phase 2 clinical trial of DBS for the treatment of TS is currently underway at the University of California, San Francisco.
- A Phase 1 clinical trial of TMS for the treatment of TS is currently underway at the University of South Florida.
- A Phase 2 clinical trial of a new type of neurostimulation called responsive neurostimulation (RNS) for the treatment of TS is currently underway at the NeuroPace headquarters in Mountain View, California.

RNS is a type of neurostimulation that uses a surgically implanted device to monitor the brain for abnormal electrical activity and deliver electrical stimulation to prevent tics. RNS has been shown to be effective in reducing the symptoms of Tourette syndrome in some patients.

The results of these clinical trials will help to determine whether neurostimulation is a safe and effective treatment option for TS.

What are the potential new treatments for TS?

In addition to the gene therapy and neurostimulation treatments mentioned above, there are a number of other potential new treatments for TS that are currently being investigated. These include

Cannabinoids Cannabinoids are chemicals found in the cannabis plant. Some studies have shown that cannabinoids can be effective in reducing the symptoms of TS. However, more research is needed to confirm these findings and to determine the long-term safety and efficacy of cannabinoids for TS.

Glutamatergic agents Glutamate is a neurotransmitter that plays a role in many brain functions, including tic suppression. Some studies have shown that glutamatergic agents, such as D-serine and riluzole, can be effective in reducing the symptoms of TS. More research is needed to confirm these findings and to determine the long-term safety and efficacy of glutamatergic agents for TS.

Psychedelic drugs Psychedelic drugs, such as psilocybin and LSD, are substances that alter perception and mood. Some studies have shown that psychedelic drugs can be effective in reducing the symptoms of a variety of mental health conditions, including TS. However, more research is needed to confirm these findings and to determine the long-term safety and efficacy of psychedelic drugs for TS.

Immune-based therapies Some scientists believe that TS may be caused by an autoimmune reaction. As a result, some researchers are investigating the use of immune-based therapies to treat TS. Immune-based therapies work by suppressing the immune system. Some studies have shown that immune-based therapies can be effective in reducing the symptoms of TS. However, more research is needed to confirm these findings and to determine the long-term safety and efficacy of immune-based therapies for TS.

It is important to note that all of these potential new treatments for TS are still in the early stages of development. More research is needed to determine their safety and efficacy. However, the results of existing studies suggest that there is a lot of promise for new and innovative treatments for TS in the future.

What is the outlook for people with TS?

The outlook for people with Tourette Syndrome (TS) can vary depending on the severity of their symptoms and the impact they have on their daily lives. However, with appropriate treatment and support, many people with TS are able to manage their symptoms and lead fulfilling lives.

It is important to note that TS is a chronic condition, meaning that it cannot be cured, but it can be managed with treatment. The main goal of treatment is to reduce the severity of symptoms and improve the person's quality of life.

The following are some of the factors that can improve the outlook for people with TS:

Early diagnosis and treatment Early diagnosis and treatment can help to reduce the severity of symptoms and improve the person's quality of life.

Medications There are several medications available that can help to reduce the severity of tics and other symptoms associated with TS.

Behavioral therapy Behavioral therapy, such as habit reversal training and exposure and response prevention, can help people with TS to manage their tics and other symptoms.

Lifestyle changes Making lifestyle changes such as avoiding stress, getting enough sleep, and exercising regularly can help to reduce the severity of symptoms.

Support Having a strong support system, including family, friends, and healthcare professionals, can help people with TS to cope with the challenges of the condition.

Despite these positive factors, people with TS may still face challenges in their daily lives. They may experience social stigma, discrimination, and difficulties in their personal and professional relationships. Therefore, it is important to raise awareness and promote understanding of TS to help people with the condition to lead fulfilling lives.

Tthe outlook for people with TS is variable, but with appropriate treatment and support, many people with TS are able to manage their symptoms and lead fulfilling lives. It is important to raise awareness and promote understanding of TS to help people with the condition to overcome the challenges they face.

Common Challenges Faced by People with TS

1. **Social Stigma** Individuals with Tourette Syndrome (TS) often face social stigma and misconceptions about their condition, leading to misunderstandings and isolation.

2. **Bullying and Teasing** Children and adults with TS may experience bullying and teasing due to their tics, leading to emotional distress and low self-esteem.

3. **Educational Challenges** TS symptoms can interfere with concentration and learning, posing challenges in educational settings. Students may struggle with attention, writing, or disruptive tics.

4. **Employment Discrimination** Some individuals with TS face discrimination in the workplace, affecting their job opportunities and career growth. Employers may not understand the condition or may have misconceptions about it.

5. **Anxiety and Depression** TS is often accompanied by anxiety and depression, which can significantly impact mental health and daily functioning. The stress of managing tics and the emotional toll of social stigma contribute to these mental health challenges.

6. **Social Relationships** Difficulties in social interactions can strain relationships, making it challenging to maintain friendships and romantic partnerships. The involuntary nature of tics can lead to misunderstandings and discomfort.

Habit Reversal Training (HRT) and Exposure and Response Prevention (ERP)

1. **Habit Reversal Training (HRT)** HRT is a behavioral therapy technique used to manage tics. It involves identifying the urges or sensations preceding tics and learning competing responses to replace the tic behavior. The individual practices these responses to gain control over their tics.

2. **Exposure and Response Prevention (ERP)** ERP is a cognitive-behavioral therapy (CBT) technique commonly used to treat obsessive-compulsive disorder (OCD) but can also be applied to TS. It involves exposing individuals to situations that trigger their tics or obsessive thoughts (exposure) and then preventing the usual response (response prevention). Over time, this helps reduce the intensity and frequency of tics or obsessive behaviors.

Raising Awareness and Promoting Understanding of TS

1. **Educational Events** Organize workshops, seminars, or webinars about TS in your community. Invite experts, psychologists, or neurologists to speak and answer questions.

2. **School Presentations** Offer to give presentations about TS in local schools to educate students, teachers, and staff. Providing accurate information can reduce stigma and promote understanding.

3. **Social Media Campaigns** Utilize social media platforms to share informative posts, videos, and personal stories related to TS. Engage

with TS advocacy organizations and use relevant hashtags to reach a broader audience.

4. **Community Support Groups** Establish or participate in local TS support groups where individuals and families can share experiences, offer support, and learn from one another.

5. **Collaborate with Schools** Work with schools to create a supportive environment for students with TS. Provide resources to teachers and classmates to foster understanding and empathy.

6. **Media Engagement** Write articles, blogs, or op-eds about TS and submit them to local newspapers or online platforms. Positive media coverage can raise awareness and challenge stereotypes.

7. **Participate in TS Awareness Events** Support and participate in TS awareness events organized by advocacy organizations. These events often provide opportunities to connect with others and amplify your advocacy efforts.

By raising awareness, promoting understanding, and providing accurate information about TS, you can contribute to a more inclusive and supportive community for individuals living with the condition.

Conclusion

Summary of key points

Tourette Syndrome (TS) is a neurodevelopmental disorder characterized by multiple motor tics and at least one vocal tic.

TS is often associated with other conditions, such as attention deficit hyperactivity disorder (ADHD), obsessive-compulsive disorder (OCD), and anxiety disorders.

The exact cause of TS is not known, but it is believed to involve a combination of genetic and environmental factors.

There is no cure for TS, but various treatments can help manage the symptoms.

Behavioral therapy, such as habit reversal training and exposure and response prevention, can be effective in reducing tics.

Medications, such as dopamine blockers and antipsychotics, can also be used to reduce tics.

Deep brain stimulation is a surgical procedure that has been shown to be effective in reducing tics in some people with TS.

It is important to raise awareness and promote understanding of TS in order to reduce stigma and improve the lives of people with TS.

Tourette Syndrome (TS) is a complex and multifaceted neurodevelopmental disorder that affects a significant number of individuals worldwide. Characterized by the presence of multiple motor tics and at least one vocal tic, TS can have a profound impact on an individual's quality of life, social interactions, and daily functioning.

While the exact cause of TS is still not fully understood, research has made significant strides in identifying the underlying genetic and environmental factors that contribute to its development. The role of genetics, the impact of stress and anxiety, and the involvement of various brain regions all play a critical role in shaping the expression of TS symptoms.

Despite the challenges posed by TS, there is hope for individuals affected by the disorder. A range of treatments, including behavioral therapy, medication, and deep brain stimulation, can help manage symptoms and improve quality of life. Moreover, advocacy efforts and increased awareness have helped to reduce stigma and promote greater understanding of TS.

However, there is still much work to be done. Further research is needed to better understand the underlying mechanisms of TS, to develop more effective treatments, and to address the significant unmet needs of individuals affected by the disorder. Additionally, greater awareness and education are necessary to combat stigma and promote greater understanding of TS among the general public, healthcare professionals, and educators.

Ultimately, TS is a complex and multifaceted disorder that requires a comprehensive and interdisciplinary approach to management and treatment. By working together to advance research, promote awareness, and improve access to care, we can help ensure that individuals with TS are able to reach their full potential and live fulfilling lives.